T0235079

Register Now for Online Access
to Your Book!

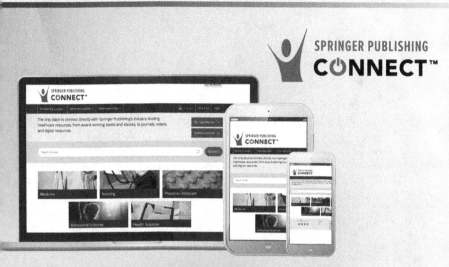

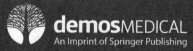

Physical Medicine and Rehabilitation Oral Board Review

Interactive Case Discussions

Second Edition

Editor

R. Samuel Mayer, MD, MEHP
Associate Professor and Vice Chair of Education
Department of Physical Medicine and Rehabilitation
Johns Hopkins University School of Medicine;
Director, Inpatient Hospital
Johns Hopkins Hospital
Baltimore, Maryland

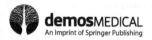

demosMEDICAL
An Imprint of Springer Publishing

Copyright © 2021 Springer Publishing Company, LLC
Demos Medical Publishing is an imprint of Springer Publishing Company.

Springer Publishing Company, LLC
11 West 42nd Street, New York, NY 10036
www.springerpub.com
connect.springerpub.com/

Acquisitions Editor: Beth Barry
Compositor: Diacritech

ISBN: 978-0-8261-7751-3
ebook ISBN: 978-0-8261-7752-0
DOI: 10.1891/9780826177520

21 22 23 24 25 / 5 4 3 2 1

Medicine is an ever-changing science. Research and clinical experience are continually expanding our knowledge , in particular our understanding of proper treatment and drug therapy. The authors, editors, and publisher have made every effort to ensure that all information in this book is in accordance with the state of knowledge at the time of production of the book. Nevertheless, the authors, editors, and publisher are not responsible for any errors or omissions or for any consequence from application of the information in this book and make no warranty, expressed or implied, with respect to the content of this publication. Every reader should examine carefully the package inserts accompanying each drug and should carefully check whether the dosage schedules therein or the contraindications stated by the manufacturer differ from the statements made in this book. Such examination is particularly important with drugs that are either rarely used or have been newly released on the market.

Library of Congress Control Number: 2021902964

Printed in the United States of America.

Contents

Contributors

Matthew N. Bartels, MD, MPH
Professor and Chair
The Arthur S. Abramson Department of Physical Medicine and Rehabilitation
Albert Einstein College of Medicine
Montefiore Health System
The Bronx, New York

Bryt A. Christensen, MD
Interventional Pain Physician
Southwest Spine and Pain Center
St. George, Utah

Tae Hwan Chung, MD
Assistant Professor
Departments of Physical Medicine and Rehabilitation and Neurology
Johns Hopkins University School of Medicine
Baltimore, Maryland

Brad E. Dicianno, MD
Associate Professor
Vice Chair for Research
Assistant Dean for Medical Student Research
Department of Physical Medicine and Rehabilitation
University of Pittsburgh School of Medicine;
Medical Director and COO
Human Engineering Research Laboratories
VA Pittsburgh Healthcare System
Pittsburgh, Pennsylvania

George Forrest, MD
Professor
Department of Rehabilitation Medicine
Albany Medical College
Albany, New York

Benjamin J. Friedman, MD
Assistant Professor
Department of Physical Medicine and Rehabilitation
Northwestern University Feinberg School of Medicine
Shirley Ryan AbilityLab
Chicago, Illinois

Joel Frontera, MD
Assistant Professor
Residency Program Director
Vice Chair for Education
Department of Physical Medicine and Rehabilitation
UTHealth Science Center
Houston, Texas

Richard L. Harvey, MD
Professor
Department of Physical Medicine and Rehabilitation
Northwestern University Feinberg School of Medicine;
Clinical Chair, Brain Innovation Center
Shirley Ryan AbilityLab
Chicago, Illinois

Deena Hassaballa, DO
Assistant Professor
Department of Physical Medicine and Rehabilitation
Northwestern University Feinberg School of Medicine;
Attending Physician
Brain Injury Medicine and Rehabilitation Program
Shirley Ryan AbilityLab
Chicago, Illinois

Sarah A. Korth, MD
Clinical Director
Keelty Center for Spina Bifida and Related Conditions
Kennedy Krieger Institute;
Attending Physician
Department of Physical Medicine and Rehabilitation
Johns Hopkins Hospital
Baltimore, Maryland

Brian J. Krabak, MD, MBA
Clinical Professor
Department of Rehabilitation Medicine
University of Washington
Seattle, Washington

Brian C. Liem, MD, FAAPMR
Clinical Assistant Professor
Department of Rehabilitation Medicine
University of Washington
Seattle, Washington

Melinda S. Loveless, MD
Clinical Assistant Professor
Department of Rehabilitation Medicine
University of Washington
Seattle, Washington

Michael Mallow, MD
Associate Professor
Residency Program Director
Department of Rehabilitation Medicine
Sidney Kimmel Medical College at Thomas Jefferson University
Philadelphia, Pennsylvania

Michael H. Marino, MD
Attending Physiatrist
Director of Disorders of Consciousness
MossRehab at Elkins Park
Elkins Park, Pennsylvania

R. Samuel Mayer, MD, MEHP
Associate Professor and Vice Chair of Education
Department of Physical Medicine and Rehabilitation
Johns Hopkins University School of Medicine;
Director, Inpatient Hospital
Johns Hopkins Hospital
Baltimore, Maryland

Andrew Nava, MD
Assistant Professor
Department of Physical Medicine and Rehabilitation
Johns Hopkins University School of Medicine
Baltimore, Maryland

Miriam Segal, MD
Attending Physiatrist
Fellowship Program Director
Drucker Brain Injury Center
MossRehab at Elkins Park
Elkins Park, Pennsylvania

Julie K. Silver, MD
Associate Professor
Associate Chair
Department of Physical Medicine and Rehabilitation
Harvard Medical School and Spaulding Rehabilitation Hospital
Boston, Massachusetts

Argyrios Stampas, MD
Assistant Professor
Department of Physical Medicine and Rehabilitation
McGovern Medical School
UTHealth Science Center
Houston, Texas

Heikki Uustal, MD
Medical Director
Prosthetic/Orthotic Team
Attending Physiatrist
JFK Johnson Rehabilitation Institute
Edison, New Jersey;
Associate Clinical Professor
Physical Medicine and Rehabilitation
Rutgers–Robert Wood Johnson Medical School
Piscataway, New Jersey

Thomas K. Watanabe, MD
Clinical Director
Drucker Brain Injury Center
MossRehab at Elkins Park
Elkins Park, Pennsylvania

Amanda Wise, DO
Resident Physician
Department of Rehabilitation Medicine
University of Washington
Seattle, Washington

Introduction

Physical medicine and rehabilitation (PM&R) is one of the broadest and most challenging specialties in medicine. Physiatrists see patients of all age groups with impairments of every organ system and must have a keen understanding of anatomy, biomechanics, ergonomics, exercise physiology, kinesiology, neurophysiology, pharmacology, and psychology. They not only prescribe medications and perform procedures, but also prescribe prosthetics, orthotics, splints, and complex medical equipment. They lead interdisciplinary teams that address the holistic bio-psycho-social and spiritual needs of people with disabling conditions. No wonder board certification preparation becomes a daunting task for examinees.

ABOUT THE EXAM

In PM&R, board certification has three components: The first component, Part I, is a written examination testing medical knowledge; the second component, Part II, is an oral examination that tests clinical practice skills. The third component, Part III, is maintenance of certification (MOC), which is an ongoing educational and evaluation process after attainment of initial certification. Part I is taken in August after completion of residency training. Nine months later (in May), examinees can take Part II after they've passed Part I and gained some experience in clinical practice or fellowship. The final component is ongoing MOC, which promotes lifelong learning.

The Part I exam focuses on knowledge. The knowledge base for PM&R has enormous breadth and depth. However, the process of studying for a knowledge-based test should be familiar to most physicians. There are a host of textbooks, several board review books, and a number of question banks available to hone one's familiarity with the field. Part II, on the other hand, tests skills and behaviors. The Accreditation Committee for Graduate Medical Education (ACGME) defined six core competencies for physicians: medical knowledge, clinical care, practice-based learning, communication, professionalism, and systems-based practice. Part I tests the first of these competencies, while Part II tests the remainder.

The American Board of Physical Medicine and Rehabilitation (ABPMR) made some adjustments in the Part II examination in 2020. Due to COVID-19, the examination is being conducted remotely using a tele-video platform. There is some possibility this platform may continue indefinitely, as it saves considerable travel expenses. The exam consists of two examination sessions, each 50 minutes in duration, with two different examiners. The exam is divided into five domains:

 Domain A: Data Acquisition: This domain is used to evaluate the acquisition of data that is critical to the provision of quality patient care. The appropriateness of the critical data identified by the candidate should be reflected in this rating. This includes history, physical exam, and psychosocial situation. Rather than responding to the examinee by answering their questions (as in previous exams), the examiner will have the examinee explain their approach to obtaining the history and physical. The examiner may ask why an examinee would want to know that data. The pertinent data will be provided at the conclusion of this domain to enable the examinee to proceed to the next domain.

Domain B: Problem-Solving: This domain addresses the appropriateness of the candidate's organization of data collection activities in relation to patient management decisions. The components of this domain include the integration of medical knowledge and acquired data to prioritize rehabilitation goals and generate a differential diagnosis. The examinee should demonstrate the ability to utilize evidence-based medicine, information technology, and research and statistical tools to answer questions in this domain.

Domain C: Patient Management: This domain addresses patient treatment decisions and the sequence of management actions. The components of this domain include the prescription of medications, exercises, modalities, equipment, and injections. The examinee will be expected to describe a comprehensive treatment plan including patient monitoring and follow-up, as well as prevention of complications and promotion of health and function.

Domain D: Systems-Based Practice: This domain addresses the candidate's ability to operate within the healthcare system to supplement patient management. The components of this domain include knowledge of the healthcare delivery system, justification of resource use, and appropriate use of referrals. The examinee should demonstrate the ability to evaluate outcomes, benefits, risks, and costs in the provision of care.

Domain E: Interpersonal and Communication Skills: This domain rates the demonstrated concern, knowledge, and skill of the candidate in dealing with the patient's questions and concerns, as well as with the concerns of the patient's family. The components of this domain include communication with patients, families, and rehabilitation team members. The examinee should demonstrate listening skills, empathy, respect for diversity, and inclusion. The examinee will be asked about ethics and professionalism issues.

How does one study for this? I would first advise that "studying" is the wrong approach. One attains skills by doing, not by reading about them. It takes practice, practice, practice. You will learn most from your patients; listen to them carefully as their stories will enlighten you. Next, take advantage of your mentors' skills and experience. Watch them examine patients, scoop up their pearls, and, above all, ask them questions and get their feedback. The case scenarios in this book are those encountered every day at the bedside. In general, the cases used by the ABPMR are not exotic or esoteric; they are meant to cover common problems encountered in a general physiatrist practice. The emphasis is on clinical practice, not trivial pursuit of obscure medical knowledge. You will not be asked to recite the medical literature, although it can help you to use clinical guidelines in your answers to demonstrate familiarity with evidence-based medicine. Be specific but concise in your responses. Each examiner is given 40 minutes to review three to four cases with you. The cases are standardized. You do not need to complete all of the cases to pass. Often, the last one or two cases that an examiner has to present are trial cases that the board is testing out for psychometric properties and will not be used in the actual scoring. You will have three examiners. The time schedule is rigid.

HOW TO USE THIS BOOK

This workbook is an additional tool, unique in its format. It walks the reader through cases in an interactive format. While it can be used individually, many may choose to use it with a partner or in small groups so that learners can give answers aloud, simulating the oral board exam. The cases are structured in a similar format to the ABPMR Part II. The content mirrors the exam outline, which is available on the ABPMR website. Although none of the authors are current oral examiners (this would be a conflict of interest), all are board certified and highly experienced clinicians, many with national and international reputations for excellence in their subspecialties. The exam consists of questions about case vignettes. Each vignette fits into one or more diagnostic categories (there are nine broad diagnostic categories), and each may focus on one or more evaluation or management skills. Each case tests five clinical skills: data acquisition, problem-solving, patient management, system-based practice, and interpersonal and communication skills. Each vignette in this book includes material in italics representing data provided by the examiner to the examinee with questions about each of these clinical skills.

We have used icons to code the questions to correspond to these five clinical skills: Data acquisition questions typically focus on the history and physical exam. Problem-solving frequently deals with diagnostic skills or biomechanics. Patient management includes all aspects of treatment: medication, equipment, injections, rehabilitation therapies, and referrals to other specialists, including surgery. System-based practice refers to psychosocial and economic issues; quality improvement projects may also be discussed. Communication skills will be evaluated by the examiners. Be prepared to explain things in lay terms as if you were talking to a patient.

HINTS

Here are some hints for examinees. Dress and act professionally. Dress tends to be more formal than most clinical workplaces. Men wear suits and ties; women may also wear suits or conservative skirts and blouses. Treat these case vignettes like real patients; picture the examiner as a patient in front of you. Ask open-ended questions of the examiner; get additional detail on the patient's history and physical exam. Be empathetic and sensitive in your communication, just as you would be with a real patient. Be cautious not to violate ethical standards like patient privacy and informed consent in your answers. Speak slowly and articulate clearly. Use proper grammar. Do not be self-conscious if you have an accent—we all have accents of some type. Although easier said than done, be calm and natural, confident but not cocky.

While this text is intended as a board review workbook to be used in preparation for the Part II exam, other audiences will find it helpful as well. All PM&R residents and fellows should have a copy—it is never too early to prepare for the oral exam. Residency program directors and faculty will find these cases useful in bedside and didactic instruction. Those preparing for MOC should also find this useful. Practicing clinicians can use these vignettes to hone up on skills in patient populations that they see less frequently.

R. Samuel Mayer

1 Amputations, Prosthetics, and Orthotics

Heikki Uustal

This is a 35-year-old male with a recent right below-the-knee amputation 1 week ago. You see the patient in your outpatient office setting shortly after discharge from the hospital.

Questions

1. What more do want to know about the patient's history, comorbidities, and social situation? Please tell me why you are asking for the specifics.

2. How would you go about performing a physical exam on this patient? Why are these maneuvers or exam components important?

The patient was involved in a motor vehicle accident resulting in crush injury to the right foot, requiring right below-the-knee amputation. There were no other significant injuries.

The patient is a well-developed male with normal strength and range of motion (ROM) of the upper limbs. There is right below-the-knee amputation with approximately 5 inches of bone length and moderate soft tissue coverage with bulbous shape. Surgical site is clean and dry with staples in place. ROM in the lower limbs is within functional limits and strength is at least 4/5 in the critical muscles. The patient is independent from wheelchair level but can stand and hop for household distance with crutches.

3. What is the functional prognosis for this patient?

4. What diagnostic tests would you order and why?

5. Outline the treatment plan. Please tell me the initial treatment and next steps after that.

The patient is quite concerned regarding his potential for return to work in construction. He has a high school education level and no other work experience beyond manual labor. It is unlikely he will be able to return to his previous work, and there is no obvious opportunity for sedentary or light-duty work.

6. How might the care be facilitated, or how would you address this dilemma?

The patient is married and has two young children. The wife is reporting that the patient is withdrawn from family activities and is often angry since the amputation. She is uncertain how to approach him or how to discuss this with her children.

7. Tell me in lay terms how you would approach this conversation.

Answers

1. Cause of the amputation and hospital course.

   Were multiple procedures or surgeries required?

   Were there are any other injuries or medical complications?

   Describe any pain including surgical pain, phantom limb pain, or other pain.

   Did you receive any type of physical therapy (PT) or occupational therapy (OT) prior to discharge from the hospital?

   Was any ongoing therapy ordered after discharge?

   What is your current functional status for self-care and mobility?

   What was your functional status for self-care and mobility prior to this event?

   Did you have any prior medical problems or past medical history?

   Tell me about your home environment: Are there any stairs indoors or outdoors to access the home?

   Who is home with you and are they available to provide any support?

   Were you working prior to amputation and what are your work responsibilities?

   What family responsibilities did you have previously?

   What recreational or social activities did you participate in previously?

   Were you driving prior to this event?

   Tell me your daily routine at home both now and prior to this event.

   All of this information will help to establish functional goals for the patient and help prescribe the proper prosthesis.

2. Brief cognitive assessment to ensure patient can understand and retain information and instructions. Hearing and vision assessment to ensure there are no barriers to education and training. Cardiopulmonary assessment to assess for any cardiac or pulmonary barriers or limitations to training. Examination of the amputation residual limb, including appropriate bone segment, bone length, quantity and quality of soft tissue coverage, overall shape, healing of surgical site, any open wounds, tenderness to palpation, and overall skin status. Strength examination of lower limbs, specifically the critical muscles for ambulation including bilateral hip extension and abduction, bilateral knee extension, and remaining ankle. Strength examination of upper limbs for critical muscles to use assistive device, including grip, elbow extensors, and shoulder depressors (pectoralis, latissimus dorsi). Grade 4/5 strength is required for all these critical muscles for initial ambulation. ROM at bilateral hips and knees to assess for potential flexion contractures. Sensory testing of the residual limb and remaining foot for potential risks of skin breakdown in the future. Assess the ability to independently move from sitting to standing position, maintain standing balance, and hop with assistive device if appropriate and safe.

3. This patient has traumatic right transtibial amputation from motor vehicle accident without other associated injuries or comorbidities. Functional prognosis for traumatic amputations is much better than for those with vascular amputations.

4. No further diagnostic testing is necessary at this time. However, because this is a younger individual with traumatic amputation, he is at higher risk for heterotopic bone formation in the near future. Follow-up x-ray of the residual limb within 2 to 3 months may be indicated, particularly if there are problems with prosthetic fitting or any irregularities palpated on examination.

5. The patient is ready to proceed with outpatient preprosthetic therapy program, which would include PT and OT for strengthening and ROM of upper limbs and lower limbs, safe and independent mobility with assistive device, shrinking and shaping of the residual limb with Ace wrapping, desensitizing the residual limb, education regarding prosthetic fitting and training, and a home exercise program.

   Monitor the surgical site healing and anticipate staple removal at week 3 or week 4 post-op. Once the staples are removed and the surgical site is healed, the shrinker sock can be fitted to further shape the limb and prepare for prosthetic fitting.

   Assessment of the patient's previous functional status will help to determine the patient's future functional potential with a prosthesis. The Medicare functional levels 1 to 4 are commonly used to help assign a functional status and plan the prosthetic device and componentry. The detailed prescription for the patient's prosthesis should be determined based on the patient's previous functional status and potential functional goals. The patient and prosthetist should be involved in this discussion and determination. The details of the prescription should include the specific socket design, including soft interface, suspension, socket material, pilon material, prosthetic foot, and any other supplies needed. The determination of prosthetic foot is most often based on the patient's functional level. As an example, if the patient is a functional level 3, then a dynamic response foot would be most appropriate.

   Other treatment programs would include driver training to teach the patient to use the left foot pedal for return to independent driving.

   Ongoing assessment of patient's pain status and psychological adjustment to limb loss.

   The patient should be followed on a regular basis by the rehab physician to monitor all of the earlier components of the treatment program.

6. Referral to a vocational counselor for more detailed vocational evaluation and possible retraining.

7. It is not unusual to have difficulty with adjustment to any disability, including limb loss. Some people struggle with their loss of independence and ability to perform as they did prior to amputation. This can lead to anger and withdrawal. Often professional counseling is required. I can refer you to a psychologist for further evaluation and management. There are also local support groups and peer counselors available that can help you deal with the situation.

BIBLIOGRAPHY

Cuccurullo SJ. *Physical Medicine and Rehabilitation Board Review*. 4th ed. Demos Medical; 2020.

Edelstein JE, Moroz A. *Lower-Limb Prosthetics and Orthotics: Clinical Concepts*. SLACK; 2011.

Esquenazi A. Amputation rehabilitation and prosthetic restoration. From surgery to community reintegration. *Disabil Rehabil*. 2004;26:831–836. https://doi.org/10.1080/09638280410001708850

Smith DG, Michael JW, Bowker JH. *Atlas of Amputations and Limb Deficiencies: Surgical, Prosthetic, and Rehabilitation Principles*. 3rd ed. American Academy of Orthopedic Surgeons; 2004:503–505, 541–555.

A 72-year-old male with diabetes, peripheral neuropathy, and peripheral vas-cular disease presents with recent right above-the-knee amputation (2 weeks ago) secondary to infection in the foot. PT was able to mobilize the patient to wheelchair mobility and limited hopping of up to 20 feet with a walker and supervision. His cardiovascular status now is stable, and the patient has only minimal pain, which is controlled with medications. He is currently in a sub-acute rehab facility.

Questions

1. What more do you want to know about this patient's history? What further information regarding his history or previous activity will help to predict his functional outcome?

2. How would you perform the physical exam and why?

The patient was a limited community ambulator prior to amputation and had a 6-month history of declining function due to ulcers and ischemia of the right foot. He has a right transfemoral amputation with long bone length (70% compared to opposite limb) with good soft tissue coverage and a cylinder shape. There is minimal tenderness to palpation, but there are staples in place and some drainage from the surgical site. He has hip extension only to neutral bilaterally.

3. Explain the decision-making process to determine the patient's functional potential and prosthetic fitting.

4. Is further testing needed?

The patient has an ejection fraction of 25% and mild occlusive disease in the remaining foot. The white blood cell count (WBC) is mildly elevated at 11k and hemoglobin is 10.

5. What is your treatment plan?

The wife is concerned that she cannot handle the patient at home until he can walk with a prosthesis, particularly since they have stairs to enter the house and to get up to the bedroom. She was told it would be 2 months before he can walk.

6. How would you address this problem?

Family members are recommending that both the patient and his wife move into an assisted living center and sell their house now to avoid an accident or disaster at home.

7. How would you help resolve or explain these options better in lay terms?

Answers

1. The patient's functional mobility status prior to amputation and the length of time since he last walked a significant distance are two important factors to determine his potential for future ambulation with a prosthesis. These should be explored in detail. A prolonged period of disability prior to amputation will require a longer rehabilitation program due to potential deconditioning and contractures. The patient's cardiopulmonary status, including testing for ejection fraction and history of myocardial infarction (MI) or congestive heart failure (CHF), are critical to assess the patient's potential with a prosthesis. We know the energy cost of ambulation with an above-knee prosthesis is approximately 40% to 60% higher than a similar able-bodied person at self-selected speed, and therefore places a significant demand on cardiac function. The patient's daily activity, home environment, and social support system will help determine when he can return home.

2. His muscle strength and ROM in all four limbs, in addition to his residual limb length, will influence his potential for prosthetic ambulation.

   Lower limb: Strength testing of hip extensors and hip abductors on the amputation side, in addition to knee extensors and ankle dorsiflexion/plantarflexion on the opposite side. Grade 4/5 strength in these muscles is critical to get from sit to stand and maintain stability during ambulation. With underlying neuropathy, the patient may have weakness or sensory loss in the remaining foot/ankle resulting in impaired balance or foot drop. These issues will further compromise recovery and functional potential.

   Upper limb: Strength testing of bilateral elbow extensors, shoulder depressors (pectoralis, latissimus), and grip. Grade 4/5 strength in these muscles is necessary to allow a patient to support himself with an assistive device and prevent falls. ROM at bilateral hips and knees is critical since flexion contractures are common at these levels. Hip extension of 10 to 20 degrees is essential for reciprocal gait. Examination of the residual limb for bone length, soft tissue coverage, shape, tenderness to palpation, and wound healing.

3. The patient's functional potential will be limited community ambulation, or likely less, based on the level of amputation (above the knee), previous activity, underlying medical conditions, hip contractures, and general deconditioning from prolonged disability prior to amputation. The decision on prosthetic components should be based on the Medicare functional level and your assessment of the patient:

   Level 0 = Nonambulatory

   Level 1 = Transfers or limited household ambulatory

   Level 2 = Household and limited community ambulatory

   Level 3 = Unlimited community ambulatory

   Level 4 = High energy or activity beyond normal ambulation

   If the patient is determined to be a level 2 ambulator, then the guidelines suggest a stance control knee and multiaxis foot. The socket design for transfemoral amputation is commonly an ischial containment socket with flexible inner socket and rigid frame, soft interface (gel liner, socks), and suspension with a waist belt, pin/strap attached to the gel liner or suction. The residual limb is not ready for fitting because the staples are still in place, and there is drainage from the surgical site. Concerns surrounding infection or healing may delay the prosthetic fitting significantly.

4. Understanding the patient's cardiopulmonary status and peripheral vascular status is critical to prevent further catastrophic events. Cardiac echo and arterial Doppler studies to assess vascular status may be required if he has symptoms of angina or dyspnea, or claudication in the left limb. Complete blood count (CBC) to detect early signs of infection or anemia should be considered.

5. The patient needs close monitoring of the surgical site for signs of infection and treatment with targeted antibiotics if any signs develop. Continued shrinking of the residual limb with Ace wrap and application of dressing if drainage continues. Culture of the drainage should be considered. Since the patient is currently in a subacute rehab facility, he should continue with comprehensive rehab program including strengthening and active assisted range of motion (AAROM) with cardiac monitoring to restore strength and ROM prior to prosthetic fitting. Slowly mobilizing the patient within cardiac parameters is still encouraged. Follow up with the surgeon for staple removal when indicated. If and when the surgical site heals and staples are removed, then prosthetic fitting can proceed. Prosthetic training can be completed as inpatient if there are concerns of cardiac tolerance or as outpatient with cardiac precautions.

6. If the patient has adequate insurance coverage to stay in the subacute facility for the entire prosthetic fitting and training period, then this may be ideal. However, in all likelihood, the patient will require home services, home equipment, and possibly home modifications to accommodate his needs. Providing home nursing and therapy services can be arranged by social services. A ramp for access to the home may be needed if there are steps outside. Home equipment such as a hospital bed, commode, and wheelchair may be needed to stay on the first floor. A home health aide may be needed to assist with self-care tasks.

7. Explaining the potential for falls in a home setting compared to a wheelchair accessible setting may help to make this decision easier. The access to medical or nursing assistance may also be reassuring. Maintaining independence sometimes requires a change in environment.

BIBLIOGRAPHY

Edelstein JE, Moroz A. *Lower-Limb Prosthetics and Orthotics: Clinical Concepts.* SLACK; 2011.

Esquenazi A. Amputation rehabilitation and prosthetic restoration. From surgery to community reintegration. *Disabil Rehabil.* 2004;26:831–836. https://doi.org/10.1080/09638280410001708850

Smith DG, Michael JW, Bowker JH. *Atlas of Amputations and Limb Deficiencies: Surgical, Prosthetic, and Rehabilitation Principles.* 3rd ed. American Academy of Orthopedic Surgeons; 2004:503–505, 541–555.

A 34-year-old carpenter severed his right forearm below the elbow in a work injury 3 weeks ago. He is referred to your prosthetic clinic by his trauma surgeon.

Questions

1. What further questions do you have about his history that would help you prescribe a prosthesis for him?

2. What are important key elements in the physical exam?

The limb was severed by a motorized saw. His pain is reasonably well controlled with oxycodone and naproxen. He has phantom sensations, but no phantom pain. He is right-hand dominant. He has no significant past medical history. He wants to eventually return to work as a carpenter. He enjoys hunting, fishing, and canoeing. Workers' compensation is paying for his medical care and rehabilitation after this injury. His incision is well-healed and sutures have been removed. The amputation is at 5 cm from the olecranon process (very short category). There is no point tenderness. Elbow flexion and extension strength are 4/5. He has approximately 45 degrees of pronation and supination.

3. What are the major considerations in prescribing a prosthesis for this man? What are the key components of a below-elbow (transradial) prosthesis? What special adaptations would help make the prosthesis more functional for him?

4. What diagnostic tests are indicated at this time?

5. Outline the treatment plan for the patient.

The patient is struggling with return to his previous work activities as a finish carpenter for a construction company. He is afraid he cannot keep up with the demands of the job and he will get fired.

6. How do you address this?

The patient reports that his interactions at home with his wife and 1-year-old daughter are strained because he is afraid to handle his daughter, thinking he might hurt her with the prosthesis. This is leading to some arguments with his wife.

7. In lay terms, tell me how you would help resolve this.

Answers

1. What was the nature of the injury and the treatment? Were there other injuries or surgeries? How did he do after surgery regarding mobility and self-care? Does he have any open wounds? How was his pain treated? How is his surgical pain now, and does he have phantom pain? Did he receive PT or OT post-op? Is he tolerating Ace wrap or compression of the residual limb? Describe his daily activities before the injury. What are his vocational and recreational goals? Hand dominance? Any previous medical history or injury?

2. Start the exam on the opposite upper limb to establish a baseline of strength, ROM, and coordination at shoulder, elbow, and hand. As you examine the involved limb, check the scapulothoracic ROM and strength in addition to glenohumeral ROM and strength. This may be critical for body-powered prosthetic control. Check elbow ROM and strength, then pronation and supination of the forearm. Establish the bone length of the residual limb and the soft tissue coverage. How is the incision healing? Any tenderness to palpation? Can he still contract residual limb muscles for potential use with myoelectric control prosthesis?

3. He wishes to return to manual labor and outdoor sports activities. A manually powered prosthesis may be more durable and reliable for these conditions. His residual limb is short, and that will require some adaptation to the suspension (likely a harness). Because he has limited supination and pronation, his prosthetic wrist should allow for manual pronation/supination positioning. The prosthetic hand can be myoelectrically powered or body-powered. The latter may be more practical for him if he intends to use it in wet conditions or for heavier activities. Body-powered terminal devices (hooks or hands) can be voluntary opening or voluntary closing devices. Voluntary opening devices are easier to use, particularly for prolonged grasp, but voluntary closing devices can apply more force or be used for finer movements. The prosthetic wrist can have friction control of supination and pronation, which may rotate to supination during heavier lifting. Because his limb is short, he will likely need a harness suspension, as self-suspension with a supracondylar sleeve or wedge may not hold his prosthesis in place adequately. A figure 8 harness has additional suspension straps compared to a figure 9 harness. The patient may also be a candidate for a myoelectric control prosthesis for social or light duty activity. Assessing the myoelectric signal from the residual limb muscles is essential to insure he can control the terminal device properly.

4. No diagnostic tests are necessary now. If he had point tenderness or palpable masses in the residual limb, a forearm x-ray to look for bony fragments, foreign objects, or heterotopic bone formation could be considered.

5. If the surgical site is healed and the limb shape is tapered, he may be ready to proceed with prosthetic fitting and training. Detailed prosthetic prescription

as outlined earlier is provided, and the process of prosthetic fitting and training is explained to the patient. Many patients require both PT and OT programs for upper limb prosthetic training to focus on different activities for self-care and potential return to work. The therapy program can be outpatient 3x/week for 4 weeks, and he should be reassessed at that time. Return to all previous activities, including driving, should be considered. He will need to learn cross-dominance since fine motor skills will still be better on the left hand. Assess for psychological adjustment to limb loss and change in body image on every visit to avoid depression or withdrawal. The prosthetic team should continue to follow the patient long term for continued functional assessment and problems. The patient may be eligible for other prosthetic devices for different settings, and these should be explored. There are a variety of terminal devices that are designed for work activities (tools), recreational activities (fishing, hunting, canoeing), or for home activities (kitchen utensils) that connect directly to the prosthesis.

6. Because this is a work-related injury, his employer needs to make reasonable accommodations for his return to work. If this is not possible, then retraining for a different job may be required. He can be referred to a vocational counselor for assessment and retraining. He should be discussing this with his case manager also.

7. Some of this can be resolved with careful practice and patience. Patients often lose their patience quickly because of other underlying psychological stresses from the amputation. Referral to psychology services for some ongoing counseling for the patient and his wife may be helpful. Reassurance from medical professionals that he will be able to help with his daughter's care helps, but sometimes meeting with other patients or families with similar issues is even more helpful. Amputee support groups may also be valuable to get peer group support in these daily activities.

BIBLIOGRAPHY

Edelstein JE, Moroz A. *Lower-Limb Prosthetics and Orthotics: Clinical Concepts.* SLACK; 2011.
Esquenazi A. Amputation rehabilitation and prosthetic restoration. From surgery to community reintegration. *Disabil Rehabil.* 2004;26:831–836. https://doi.org/10.1080/09638280410001708850
Smith DG, Michael JW, Bowker JH. *Atlas of Amputations and Limb Deficiencies: Surgical, Prosthetic, and Rehabilitation Principles.* 3rd ed. American Academy of Orthopedic Surgeons; 2004:503–505, 541–555.
Uustal H, Meier RH 3rd. Pain issues and treatment of the person with an amputation. *Phys Med Rehabil Clin N Am.* February 2014;25(1):45–52. https://doi.org/10.1016/j.pmr.2013.09.008

A 72-year-old patient presents for evaluation of left foot drop 9 days following coronary artery bypass surgery. The patient only noticed the weakness in PT as he tried to progress his ambulation following surgery. He is currently on the rehabilitation unit and must be an independent ambulator to return home.

Questions

1. What further information would you like to know about the patient's past medical history and recent surgical history?

2. How would you perform a focused physical examination to establish the cause of the left foot drop?

The patient history is significant for underlying diabetes with peripheral neuropathy and peripheral vascular disease, hypertension, and coronary artery disease. Based on patient history, he reports no muscle weakness prior to his cardiac surgery but he did have numbness in both legs from peripheral neuropathy. He denies any previous history of back injury or neurological deficit causing left leg weakness or foot drop. On physical examination today he has only trace movements for left ankle dorsiflexion and eversion, but 4/5 strength for plantarflexion and inversion. Proximal muscles that the left hip and left knee are all 4/5 but limited somewhat by pain. There is no focal weakness in the right lower limb. He has diminished sensation in both legs below the knee to pinprick, but absent sensation on dorsum of left foot. He has fluctuating edema in both lower limbs, which is not well controlled. The patient has evidence of recent vein harvest surgical sites extending from proximal to distal on the left leg.

3. What is your working diagnosis based on history and exam, and is there any further testing necessary to confirm the diagnosis?

4. Outline the treatment plan for rehabilitation for this patient including especially orthotic management of the left foot drop to restore safe functional mobility. Explain the rationale for your choice of orthotic device and design.

The patient asks you if there is a charge for the brace since his finances are limited. If the brace is expensive, and he must pay for it, he will refuse.

5. How would you respond to this?

The patient is resistant to agree to the brace because it looks old-fashioned and heavy. He is questioning why a lighter and more modern brace cannot be used.

6. In lay terms, how would you explain the risks and benefits of various brace designs and the reason for your choice of the current brace?

Answers

1. The patient's past medical history is important to assess for any predisposing cause for weakness or other neurological problems. Specific line of questioning regarding peripheral neuropathy, back injury that may result in radiculopathy, or other neurological causes for weakness. Careful review of the surgical report and consulting with the surgeon regarding the possibility of peripheral nerve injury during surgery or perioperative period. Questioning the patient regarding any falls or other injury since surgery that may have caused compression of the left sciatic nerve or other peripheral nerves resulting in foot drop. Questioning regarding sensory loss in the lower limbs, both before surgery and after surgery, which may indicate the timing or level of nerve injury.

2. Start with cognitive assessment to ensure there is no central neurological insult such as cerebrovascular accident (CVA). It should be followed by careful neurological examination of all four limbs for strength, sensation, and tone. If there is weakness at the left ankle involving primarily the L4-L5 muscles resulting in foot drop, then proximal L4-L5 muscles should also show some weakness if radiculopathy is suspected. If there is only distal muscle weakness without proximal weakness, then peroneal nerve injury is more likely. Inspection of the surgical sites on the leg for vein harvesting as a potential source for peripheral nerve injury. Sensory testing will also provide some insight to the etiology of foot drop. If the peroneal nerve is the primary source, then sensory deficit should be isolated to the dorsum of the foot. However, this may be difficult to assess if there is underlying peripheral neuropathy causing sensory deficit bilaterally. Assessment of muscle tone should help to distinguish between upper motor neuron and lower motor neuron insult. Inspection for edema is important to start preparing for orthotic prescription to control left foot drop. Left ankle ROM, particularly for dorsiflexion, will also be important for orthotic planning.

3. Based on the history and physical exam findings, the current working diagnosis would be peripheral nerve injury, most likely to the left sciatic or peroneal nerve. The actual cause of the injury could be direct damage to the nerve during vein harvesting on the left leg or compression neuropathy as a result of positioning of the left limb during surgery or perioperatively. Without evidence of proximal muscle weakness, higher level of nerve injury is less likely. Definitive diagnosis could be established with electromyography (EMG) and nerve conduction testing. However, the patient is only 9 days since surgery and the likely onset of this injury, and EMG testing is most reliable 14 days or more after nerve injury. In addition, the patient is fully anticoagulated at present and this is a relative contraindication to EMG testing.

4. The treatment plan should continue with PT and OT for strengthening of all four limbs with cardiac precautions, AAROM, progressive ambulation, and assessment of self-care skills. The patient will require a left ankle-foot orthosis (AFO) to control left foot drop and left ankle instability during ambulation.

Because the symptoms have persisted beyond 7 days, it is unlikely that the nerve injury is neuropraxia; therefore, delayed recovery is anticipated. The patient will require a left AFO to return home safely. The choice of AFO design is dictated by the patient's muscle weakness, muscle tone, sensory status, skin integrity, and ROM at the ankle. In this case, the patient has uncontrolled edema and impaired sensation at the left foot and ankle, in addition to under-lying peripheral vascular disease and recent surgery to the left lower limb vein harvesting. Therefore, the selection of material and design that is most appropriate would be a double metal upright AFO with calf band and Velcro closure, posterior channel ankle joint with spring-assisted dorsiflexion, and solid stirrup attached to extra-depth diabetic shoe with custom-molded foot orthotic. This would allow minimal contact to the skin and minimize the risk of skin breakdown or pressure due to fluctuating edema. It also provides some adjustability at the ankle and maximum protection for the foot due to the underlying diabetes. The intimate fit of a custom plastic AFO is con-tra-indicated due to the edema and vein harvest surgical site. An off the shelf carbon fiber AFO is also less desirable due to the lack of adjustability.

5. Insurance coverage for durable medical equipment such as bracing during an inpatient hospital stay is based on the type of insurance and the medical necessity. If the patient has Medicare coverage, then bracing is allowed and covered in preparation for discharge within the last 2 days of hospitalization. However, if it is prescribed earlier in the hospital stay, the hospital is respon-sible for providing that brace under their cost and cannot charge the patient. If the patient has commercial insurance, then a prescription should be written and submitted for authorization prior to fabrication. Medical necessity for the brace should be documented and established by the ordering physician in the hospital chart.

6. Careful explanation in common terms about the increased contact to the skin with other brace designs, such as custom molded plastic AFO or even carbon fiber AFO, and the potential risk of skin irritation or breakdown. Because of the fluctuating edema, the shape of the leg will constantly be changing from morning to evening or day to day, and therefore minimal contact to the leg is required. The soft contact of a diabetic shoe and insert will be more protec-tive of the patient's foot due to lack of sensation compared to the more rigid contact of plastic or carbon fiber material. Finally, the adjustability of a metal brace will be an advantage if the patient's condition improves or deteriorates significantly.

BIBLIOGRAPHY

Cuccurullo SJ. *Physical Medicine and Rehabilitation Board Review.* 4th ed. Demos Medical; 2020.
Shin MR, Morozova O, Rubin J. Upper and lower limb orthoses and therapeutic footwear. AAPMR Knowledge NOW.
   https://now.aapmr.org/upper-and-lower-limb-orthoses-and-therapeutic-footwear

2 Brain Impairments and Central Nervous System Disorders

Michael H. Marino, Miriam Segal, and Thomas K. Watanabe

CASE 1

A 22-year-old female suffered respiratory and circulatory arrest secondary to status asthmaticus. She was resuscitated by emergency medical service and subsequently hospitalized for 4 weeks with multiple complications including ventilator-dependent respiratory failure requiring tracheostomy and gastrostomy tube placement. After being weaned from the ventilator, it is apparent that she has severe neurologic impairment. You are asked to see her to determine if she is a candidate for inpatient brain injury rehabilitation.

Questions

1. What are the key elements that you would like to obtain regarding this patient's history? Explain why these elements are important.

2. What are the important features upon which you would focus your physical exam and why?

The patient is awake and breathing spontaneously on humidified oxygen via tracheostomy collar. Vital signs are normal.

3. What diagnostic tests or assessments would you want to order or review?

MRI shows no focal lesions, and the EEG shows generalized slowing but no epileptiform activity. The patient's level of consciousness is very impaired at this point, and the question of prognosis has come up in order for the medical team to determine the most appropriate disposition and for appropriate counseling of the family.

4. What are the key prognostic indicators?

She is able to track the examiner and follow some simple commands, but her responses are slow. She is not vocalizing due to the tracheostomy tube but is able to mouth some words.

5. Outline your treatment plan.

The parents are seeking legal guardianship for the patient. They bring in a form from their attorney, which asks whether the patient has capacity.

6. How might you determine if this patient has capacity? What questions would you go about asking her?

Four months later, you see the patient for an outpatient visit. She was discharged from inpatient rehabilitation and then completed a course of outpatient physical therapy (PT), occupational therapy (OT), and speech therapy. She is able to walk without assistance and is performing basic activities of daily living on her own, but her family is still providing 24-hour supervision and they manage her appointments and finances. They note that sometimes they still need to cue her for safety or to complete a task. She would very much like to go back to school and resume driving and is eager to regain her independence, but her parents are anxious.

7. What are your recommendations at this point? How do you balance her goals for increased independence with her parents' concerns for safety?

Answers

1. In patients with hypoxic brain injury (HBI), a complete history includes a detailed hospital course, injury mechanism, duration of hypoxia/ischemia, duration of disordered consciousness and posthypoxic amnesia, residual impairments, and medical comorbidities thus far. These elements of the history are all important in terms of present medical stability and functional prognosis. In terms of premorbid history, it is important to obtain prior functional status (including vocational history and driving), level of education, previous history of drug or alcohol abuse, previous psychiatric history, and premorbid personality, as well as social support. This information will be important for goal setting and for contextualizing the present functional status.

2. Arousal, visual tracking, response to tactile or painful stimulation, ability to follow verbal commands, ability to accurately indicate yes/no responses, passive and active range of motion in the limbs to evaluate for spasticity, contracture, or heterotopic ossification. In patients who can participate further, the following should also be assessed: cerebellar and fine motor testing, coordination, visual testing (including testing for agnosia), orientation, attention, processing speed, memory, judgment, insight, affect, and behavior.

3. MRI will help determine if there are focal lesions from watershed infarcts. EEG may help determine any seizure activity or focal slowing.

4. In patients with severely impaired consciousness after cardiopulmonary resuscitation, appropriate functional prognostication is critical. Absent pupillary or corneal reflexes, or absent extensor motor responses 3 days after cardiac arrest, indicate an outcome that is invariably poor (Level A, strong evidence). A poor prognosis is also conferred if there is myoclonic status epilepticus within the first day (Level B, good evidence), bilaterally absent N20 response by day 3, or serum neuron-specific enolase (NSE) levels >33 mcg/L at days 1 to 3 (Level B, good evidence). Prognosis cannot be based on circumstances of cardiopulmonary resuscitation, elevated temperature, EEG, intracranial pressure, or neuroimaging studies. For patients who are comatose and in whom the initial cardiac rhythm is either ventricular tachycardia or fibrillation after cardiac arrest, therapeutic hypothermia (32–34°C for 24 hours) is highly likely to be effective in improving neurologic outcome and survival (Level A evidence).

5. Initiate a multidisciplinary rehabilitation program to promote physical and cognitive recovery. This should include attention to sleep–wake cycle, management of any agitation, tracheostomy tube weaning, management of any posthypoxic seizures or movement disorders, spasticity management and serial examinations to exclude new pathology, or improvement to guide the rehabilitation program. Rehabilitation nursing involvement is important to care for skin and for bowel and bladder management as well as to help maintain the therapeutic milieu and advance team goals. PT is important for

functional mobility and may address spasticity or dyskinesias as well. OT may introduce adaptive strategies for visual and cognitive deficits as well as self-care skills. Speech/language pathology will need to work on diet advancement as well as cognitive–linguistic deficits. A neuropsychologist can help to guide the team's efforts and provide counseling and education to the patient and family. Social work is important to coordinate transitions of care, identify resources, and keep families informed of the expected course as the patient progresses through the rehabilitation process.

6. Capacity means that the patient has adequate intellectual abilities to describe his or her medical situation, appraise alternatives, and make rational choices based on values. You might ask the patient, "Can you tell me a little bit about what happened to you and how it has effected your abilities?" You might ask what would happen if the patient did not take prescribed medications or follow through with therapies. A patient does not need to have normal intellectual function in order to have capacity.

7. Management of chronic HBI involves gradual reintegration into the community with ongoing education and support as well as appropriate referrals to community-based services. It is important to convey that gains in independence are made in a progressive manner in order to build on the patient's progress and safely restore independence in a progressive manner. The treatment may include neuropsychological (NP) evaluation and counseling or follow-up, vocational rehabilitation services, and driving evaluation if the patient is able. It is important to note that any posthypoxic seizures may affect restoration of driving privileges. You should continue to follow up to monitor for secondary conditions such as depression or other mood disturbances and refer to behavioral health as needed.

BIBLIOGRAPHY

Eslinger PJ, Zapela G, Chakara F, et al. Cognitive impairments. In: Zasler ND, et al., eds. *Brain Injury Medicine*. 2nd ed. Demos Medical; 2013:chap 51.

Geocadin RG, Wijdicks E, Armstrong MJ, et al. Practice guideline summary: reducing brain injury following cardiopulmonary resuscitation. Report of the guideline development, Dissemination, and implementation subcommittee of the American academy of neurology. *Neurology*. May 2017;88(22):2141–2149. https://doi.org/10.1212/WNL.0000000000003966

Kothari S, DiTommaso C. Prognosis after severe traumatic brain injury: a practical, evidence-based approach. In: Zasler ND, et al., eds. *Brain Injury Medicine*. 2nd ed. Demos Medical; 2013.

Sandroni C, D'Arrigo S, Nolan JP. Prognostication after cardiac arrest. *Crit Care*. 2018;22:150. https://doi.org/10.1186/s13054-018-2060-7

Wang E, Schultz B. Hypoxic brain injury. *PM&R Knowledge Now*. 2012. http://me.aapmr.org/kn/article.html?id=15

Wijdicks EFM, Hijra A, Young GB, et al. Practice parameter: prediction of outcome in comatose survivors after cardiopulmonary resuscitation (an evidence-based review). Report of the quality standards Subcommittee of the American academy of neurology. *Neurology*. 2006;6:203–210. https://doi.org/10.1212/01.wnl.0000227183.21314.cd

A 21-year-old male is being admitted to acute inpatient rehabilitation after being treated in acute care for a traumatic brain injury (TBI) and several rib fractures due to a motor vehicle crash. You are called to perform the history and physical.

Questions

1. What more do you want to know about the patient's history, comorbidities, and social situation? Please tell me why you are asking about these specifics.

2. How would you go about performing the physical exam on this patient? Why are these maneuvers/exam components important?

The records indicate that the injury occurred in a high-speed motor vehicle crash and that your patient was the driver. His initial Glasgow Coma Scale (GCS) score was 6 and his trauma workup revealed bifrontal contusions and diffuse subarachnoid hemorrhage as well as multiple rib fractures. He was intubated and sedated and had an intracranial pressure monitor placed. One week later he was extubated and transferred to a step-down floor where he had some intermittent fevers and tachycardia without an infectious source. It is now 3 weeks postinjury and he remains nonverbal. The patient is awake and appears alert. He visually tracks the examiner and pushes the examiner away when noxious stimulation is applied. His psychomotor activity is decreased. He does not follow any verbal commands or indicate any yes/no responses.

3. What is the level of severity of brain injury?

4. What formal assessment measures should be implemented on the patient and why?

The Coma Recovery Scale-Revised (CRS-R) is being used and demonstrates that this patient is in a minimally conscious state. You also note that his eye opening is frequently poor, requiring stimulation to facilitate wakefulness during therapy sessions.

5. Outline the treatment plan for this patient. Tell me the next steps if he fails to demonstrate progress.

Your patient has a fiancé who wants to be his main point of contact and medical decision-maker. His parents also want to be his primary point of contact and medical decision-makers, and they do not want any information shared with his fiancée.

6. What factors would you incorporate in addressing this ethical dilemma?

Your patient continues to demonstrate signs of minimal consciousness while being treated in your specialized program for patients with disorders of consciousness. His family members do not understand what the term disorder of consciousness means.

7. Tell me in lay terms how you would describe disorders of consciousness and the difference between the levels of consciousness.

Answers

1. Certain elements of the injury history will help to determine injury severity as well as the pattern of deficits that would be expected and the prognosis for a good recovery. These would be injury mechanism, loss of consciousness (LOC) and duration, residual impairments (especially posttraumatic amnesia [PTA]), initial GCS score, associated injuries, and postinjury complications thus far. Certain elements of the preinjury history are useful in determining the course of recovery. These would be prior functional status (including vocational history and driving), level of education, previous history of drug or alcohol abuse, previous psychiatric history, previous history of TBI, social support, and premorbid personality.

2. Important elements of a physical exam in such a case are arousal, visual tracking, response to tactile or painful stimulation, ability to follow verbal commands, ability to accurately indicate yes/no responses, orientation (if possible), passive and active range of motion in the limbs (as best as can possibly be assessed if the patient cannot follow commands), and muscle tone. These elements of the exam are important to clarify the level of severity of injury (including level of consciousness), identify any focal deficits (including language, vision, weakness, and sensory loss), and identify any comorbid conditions that will affect the course of recovery.

3. This patient has a severe TBI. The core elements in determining severity of injury include GCS, duration of LOC, and duration of PTA. Mild TBIs have GCS between 13 and 15, duration of LOC of 30 minutes or less, and the duration of PTA of less than 24 hours. Conventional neuroimaging (CT and/or MRI) is normal in mild TBI. Moderate severity injuries have GCS of 9 to 12, duration of LOC between 30 minutes and 24 hours, or duration of PTA greater than 24 hours but less than 7 days. Severe TBIs have GCS less than or equal to 8, duration of LOC of greater than 24 hours, or duration of PTA of greater than 7 days.

4. Since his level of consciousness seems to be impaired, the CRS-R can be used to predict recovery. As he emerges, the Galveston Orientation and Amnesia Test (GOAT) or the Orientation-log (O-log) can be used to assess PTA. A patient is considered emerged from PTA with a score >75 on the GOAT or >25 on the O-log for 2 consecutive days. Early predictors of recovery in TBI are duration of coma (frequently defined as the time to follow commands), duration of PTA, and age. A "good" recovery on the Disability Rating Scale is defined as little no to disability. Good recovery is unlikely if the length of the coma exceeds 14 days, if the duration of PTA exceeds 3 months, or if a person age 65 years or older sustains an injury classified as severe.

5. Patients with disorders of consciousness should be treated by a multidisciplinary rehabilitation team in specialty centers that have the training and experience to perform proper diagnostic evaluation and management and

provide accurate prognostication. In order to improve eye opening and responsiveness, a thorough review of medications should be performed. including minimizing any centrally acting, sedating medications that are unnecessary. This may include opiates, benzodiazepines, antipsychotics, and medications with anticholinergic activity. If the patient is on anticonvulsants, the need to continue them should be evaluated. A normal sleep-wake cycle should be restored. Amantadine can be instituted for this patient, as it has been shown to improve the rate of neurologic recovery in patients with disorders of consciousness of traumatic etiology. Additionally, it can help improve eye opening. If the patient fails to demonstrate progress, a more thorough workup should be performed. This workup can include EEG to rule out seizure, CT head to evaluate for rebleeding or hydrocephalus, and laboratory workup to evaluate for metabolic derangement or neuroendocrine dysfunction. Electromyography/nerve conduction study can be considered to evaluate for critical illness neuropathy or myopathy which can interfere with a patient's motor output and thus limit the ability to demonstrate command following.

6. Hospital systems and specialized programs that treat patients with disorders of consciousness should have systems in place to identify the proper next of kin to establish a medical decision-maker. This is typically a legal issue, and rules can vary from state to state. Coordination of care with social work and potentially risk management/legal department within the healthcare system is advisable. Once the medical decision-maker has been determined, it is important to ascertain from that individual who they will allow information to be shared with.

7. An individual with a disorder of consciousness has an injury to the brain that has interfered with their ability to be awake and aware of their surroundings. The levels of disorders of consciousness are coma, vegetative state (sometimes referred to as unresponsive wakefulness syndrome), and minimally conscious state. In a coma, the eyes are closed all the time and the individual is never awake. In a vegetative state, the individual has times of being awake but does not show any purposeful activity or responses to the world around them. In a minimally conscious state, the individual has periods of eye-opening and can sometimes demonstrate purposeful activity or meaningful responses to the world around them; however, it is very inconsistent.

BIBLIOGRAPHY

Giacino JT, Katz DI, Schiff ND, et al. Practice guideline update recommendations summary: disorders of consciousness. Are because of physical medicine and rehabilitation. *Neurology.* 2018;99:1699–1709. https://doi.org/10.1016/j.apmr.2018.07.001

Giacino JT, Whyte J, Nakase-Richardson R, et al. Minimum competencies recommendations for programs that provide rehabilitation services for persons with disorders of consciousness: a position statement of the American Congress of rehabilitation medicine and the National Institute on disability, independent living in rehabilitation research traumatic brain injury model systems. Are because of physical medicine and rehabilitation. *Arch Phys Med Rehabil.* June 2020;101(6):1072–1089. https://doi.org/10.1016/j.apmr.2020.01.013

Kothari S, DiTommaso C. Prognosis after severe traumatic brain injury: a practical, evidence-based approach. In: Zasler ND, et al., eds. *Brain Injury Medicine.* 2nd ed. Demos Medical; 2013.

Wolf C, McLaughlin M, Khadavi M, et al. Traumatic brain injury. *PM&R Knowledge Now.* 2015. http://me.aapmr.org/kn/article.html?id=41

CASE 3

A 48-year-old man who suffered a gunshot wound to the head is in your acute inpatient rehabilitation unit. His nurse informs you that he is more lethargic this morning with difficulty waking up.

Questions

1. What more do you want to know about the patient's history, comorbidities, and hospital course? Please tell me why you are asking for these specifics.

2. How would you go about performing the physical exam on this patient? Why are these maneuvers/exam components important?

He had a right-sided decompressive craniectomy 8 weeks ago and has left-sided hemiparesis. He had no seizures. At baseline, he was alert, responsive, and appropriate but has been progressively more lethargic over the last week. He has not had any recent infections. He slept well last night. He has not had any recent medication changes. On exam he is lethargic, requiring noxious stimulation to maintain eye-opening. He is answering questions but is slow to respond. Vitals are stable. Pupillary responses are normal. His left hemiparesis is at baseline. His craniectomy site appears slightly more tense and bulging than before. The craniectomy incision is well healed and without discharge. His lungs are clear and his heart is regular.

3. What is the differential diagnosis for this patient? Tell me the most likely diagnosis and why.

4. What diagnostic test or tests would you order and why?

His metabolic and infectious workup is negative. Routine bedside EEG does not show any seizure activity but shows focal slowing over the right cerebral hemisphere with signs of cortical irritability. CT scan of the head shows a diffusely enlarged ventricular system.

5. Outline the treatment plan. Please tell me the initial treatment and next steps if that fails.

You are concerned that this patient was declining over the course of a week before the workup was initiated.

6. Describe a quality improvement project establishing guidelines on your brain injury unit for monitoring patients for hydrocephalus.

Upon review of prior neuroimaging, your patient has a progressively enlarging hydrocephalus. You must inform the family of the diagnosis.

7. Tell me in lay terms about hydrocephalus.

Answers

1. The timeframe since the injury and initial injury severity are important to better understand the patient's trajectory of recovery. Surgical history and timeframe since surgery are important to determine the likelihood of surgical complications or infections. A history of intracranial complications such as rebleeding, seizures, or hydrocephalus should be obtained because these conditions can reoccur. The examiner should inquire about sleep pattern because sleep–wake cycle reversals are common and can cause daytime somnolence. Lastly, any recent medication changes should be noted, because medication side effects can cause change in mental status. The examiner should ask about history of infections, including urinary tract infections, because these can also cause change in mental status. History of heart disease, renal disease, or diabetes should be established. Arrhythmias, acute coronary syndrome, decompensated heart failure, or hypoglycemia can all cause change in mental status.

2. The exam should start with observation for any signs of shaking/seizure. The examiner must document level of arousal and what maneuvers are required to maintain alertness. This will establish the degree of obtundation. Pupillary responses and cranial nerve exam are important because changes in these exam elements can signify the presence of elevated intracranial pressure. Change in strength or sensation from baseline can signify a new focal neurological injury. Examination of any surgical sites is important to look for signs of infection. Evaluation of the craniectomy site is imperative. A sunken flap can indicate syndrome of the trephined/sunken flap syndrome. A bulging, tense craniectomy site can indicate elevated intracranial pressure due to edema, new bleed, infection, or hydrocephalus. Examination of the heart is required to determine there is no arrhythmia. Lung examination is important to rule out pulmonary infection.

3. Differential diagnosis includes metabolic/electrolyte disturbance, rebleed/intracranial hemorrhage, hydrocephalus, seizures, central nervous system (CNS) infection (abscess or meningitis), and urinary tract infection. The most likely diagnoses are conditions that increase intracranial pressure, because his craniectomy site is bulging and more tense. These diagnoses include hemorrhage, CNS infection, and hydrocephalus. CNS infection is less likely because he is afebrile.

4. Labs and tests would include basic metabolic panel (BMP), complete blood count (CBC) with differential, urinalysis, CT head, and EEG. BMP will evaluate for metabolic/electrolyte disturbances. CBC will evaluate for infection. CT head will look for rebleed, CNS infection, and hydrocephalus. Urinalysis is to look for urinary tract infection. EEG to look for seizures.

5. Communicating hydrocephalus is more common than noncommunicating hydrocephalus after TBI. The first step is to compare the current head

CT images to prior to imaging to determine if the ventricle size is stable or enlarging. If the ventricle size is progressively enlarging, then consultation with neurosurgery should be obtained. However, if ventricle size is stable, other diagnoses should be pursued. In this case, while there are no signs of seizure on the EEG, there are signs of cortical irritability, which can lead to seizure. Repeat EEG, prolonged EEG, or sleep-deprived EEG can increase the diagnostic yield for posttraumatic seizures.

6. Do a Plan, Do, See, Act (PDSA) cycle. Perform a literature review for identifying subpopulations at risk for developing hydrocephalus (plan). Educate staff about signs and symptoms of hydrocephalus (do). See how many hydrocephalus cases are identified in your unit over a quarter, and whether they were found early (see). Then determine if further interventions, such as order sets, are needed (act).

7. Our brain has fluid-filled spaces deep inside of it. These spaces are connected to each other and circulate a fluid called cerebrospinal fluid (CSF), also called CSF. Unfortunately, as a consequence of the brain injury, these fluid-filled spaces are becoming larger and larger. Because there is only a finite amount of room inside the skull, these expanding fluid spaces are putting pressure on the rest of the brain. This pressure on the brain is interfering with his ability to be awake and participate in rehabilitation.

BIBLIOGRAPHY

Long DF. Diagnosis and management of late intracranial complications of TBI. In: Zasler ND, et al., eds. *Brain Injury Medicine*. 2nd ed. Demos Medical; 2013:chap 44.

Wolf C, McLaughlin M, Khadavi M, et al. Traumatic brain injury. *PM&R Knowledge Now*. 2015. http://me.aapmr.org/kn/article.html?id=41

Yablon SA, Dostrow VG. Post-traumatic seizures and epilepsy. In: Zasler ND, et al., eds. *Brain Injury Medicine*. 2nd ed. Demos Medical; 2013:chap 26.

CASE 4

A 17-year-old high school female student is seen in the outpatient clinic. She was injured in a soccer game 3 days ago. She says that she is here because she was hit in the head and that she could not return to soccer until she was cleared by a doctor.

Questions

1. What history should be obtained in order to better understand her injury, risk factors for a slow recovery, and to ascertain her needs?

2. What elements of the physical examination would be appropriate for this patient?

You learn that she had momentary LOC and disorientation on the field after heading a hard-driven ball. Today she still has a headache and neck pain. She reports difficulty concentrating in class. Her Montreal Cognitive Assessment (MoCA) score is 29/30. Balance is unremarkable, as is cranial nerve examination. No focal weakness or sensory deficits are noted. Reflexes are symmetric. There is full active cervical range of motion without pain. Mild tenderness in the left frontal region where she was hit by the ball. No prior history of concussions or other brain injuries. She has a personal and family history of migraine headaches.

3. What diagnoses are you considering?

4. What diagnostic tests would you order?

Postconcussion Symptoms Scale (PCSS) score is 20, with the highest scores being for headache, sensitivity to noise, feeling slowed down, having difficulty concentrating, and feeling mentally foggy. Postinjury computerized cognitive test results have not worsened compared to preinjury scores.

5. Outline an initial treatment plan and next steps if symptoms do not resolve.

The father asks that you write a letter today that can be submitted in order to allow the student to receive extra time to take a college board test. This test is scheduled for 6 months from now.

6. How do you respond?

After you explain to the father that the student needs to follow a return to play protocol that will take at least a week, he is irate, saying that there is an important "showcase" tournament this weekend that could lead to the student receiving a college scholarship. He says that he will find another doctor who will clear her if you do not.

7. How do you respond?

Answers

1. One should get a clear history of what happened and whether the episode is likely to have caused a concussion. It will be helpful to know if there was any LOC, although one can have a concussion without this. Observations from others present (e.g., parents, trainers) can help in the understanding of mechanism and severity of injury. Amnesia, altered level of alertness, behavioral changes, fatigue, nausea, headache, and balance problems are all common symptoms. Symptoms that suggest a more significant injury, such as vomiting; focal neurological complaints, such as weakness; or worsening headaches should be identified. The symptoms can help guide the physical examination. A history of concussions, preexisting medical problems (e.g., migraine headaches), and family history can help with determining those at risk for prolonged recovery.

2. Ideally, the athlete should be examined immediately on the field for changes in orientation; alertness; cranial nerve findings; and balance, coordination, and motor deficits. However, high schools frequently do not have the resources to do this, so a comprehensive neurological examination should be done in the office when the athlete is seen by the physician. This should include cognitive, sensory, motor, and cranial nerve assessments; functional evaluation of balance; and other tests as warranted based on symptoms and related findings; for example, pain generators.

3. The primary diagnosis at this point is acute concussion. The headache may be a posttraumatic headache.

4. At this point, there is no clear indication to order other diagnostic tests. There is no role for routine imaging after sports-related concussion. A PCSS score can be utilized to assess current symptoms and track symptom resolution. If she has baseline (preinjury) computerized cognitive testing data available, repeat testing to compare results is appropriate.

5. The initial treatment plan would be to avoid worsening of symptoms. This early on, it is likely that symptoms will resolve quickly with minimal intervention. Allowing some low-intensity activity as tolerated may be helpful. This includes cognitive as well as physical activity. Monitor for tolerance and quality of academic activities. Judicious use of nonsteroidal anti-inflammatory medications for the headache may be considered. Other medications, such as a triptan, may be considered to address apparent migraine headaches, especially if these medications have helped her migraines in the past. If symptoms do not continue to resolve, or the patient is having difficulty with school, a reevaluation tailored to the symptoms is important. For instance, if a headache is the primary problem, determining the type of headache (e.g., tension, migraine) may guide further intervention. Activities that provoke symptoms should be queried. This may help identify other underlying problems such as visual or vestibular problems. A further review of preinjury symptoms or conditions that may slow symptom resolution, such as poor sleep or stress/anxiety, may be helpful.

6. Sequelae of concussions usually resolve within a few weeks and it is often helpful and reassuring to let patients and families know that. At this point, it is too early to state that accommodations will be needed 6 months from now. However, you can assure them that the need can be assessed should there be lingering problems and that you would be happy to provide a letter should it be appropriate.

7. The return to play protocol was developed to help ensure that players have fully recovered from their concussion before they return to a sport and potentially have another one. Emphasize to the parent that a second concussion sustained before a first one has resolved may lead to a much longer recovery time and that this would likely result in even more of a setback for her soccer playing and the possibility of receiving a scholarship. Reinforce that your strategy is intended to help her succeed and not to hold her back. Tell him that this return to play protocol is rather standard, and that even though they have the right to choose to go elsewhere for care, it is unlikely that this strategy will allow her to be cleared sooner and may actually slow the process as another practitioner would need to schedule her and initiate a treatment plan.

BIBLIOGRAPHY

Collins M, Iverson GL, Gaetz MB, et al. Sports related concussion. In: Zasler ND, et al., eds. *Brain Injury Medicine*. 2nd ed. Demos Medical; 2013:chap 31.

DiFazio M, Silverberg ND, Kirkwood MW, et al. Prolonged activity restriction after concussion: are we worsening outcomes? *Clin Pediatr*. 2016;55(5): 443–451. https://doi.org/10.1177/0009922815589914

Guenette JP, Shenton ME, Koerte IK. Imaging of concussion in young athletes. *Neuroimaging Clin N Am*. 2018;28(1):43–53. https://doi.org/10.1016/j.nic.2017.09.004

McCrory P, Meeuwisse W, Dvorak J, et al. Consensus statement on concussion in sport—the 5th international conference on concussion in sport held in Berlin, October 2016. *Br J Sports Med*. 2017;51(11):838–847. https://doi.org/10.1136/bjsports-2017-097878

CASE 5

A 40-year-old female is referred to your outpatient clinic by her attorney for lingering symptoms related to a motor vehicle crash 9 months prior. Primary complaints include severe headaches and poor memory.

Questions

1. What information will be helpful for your initial assessment, and why?

2. What elements of the physical examination would you focus on?

She describes the crash as being rear-ended while she was stationary. The other vehicle struck her at about 15 mph. She had no LOC and took herself to the ED, where she had a GCS score of 15 and an unremarkable head CT. She insists that she never had headaches or cognitive problems before the crash but does report being treated pharmacologically for anxiety for the past 5 years. Headaches are dull, band-like, and without nausea or photophobia. She has not slept well since the crash. She is guarded when moving her head and neck, with diffuse tenderness in the cervical spine with worsening of headache complaints during this exam. Short-term memory is unremarkable and she has very good recall of the accident and time course of her symptoms. Digit span is five numbers forward and three numbers backward. She has some difficulty calculating simple change. Extraocular movements are unremarkable.

3. What diagnoses are you entertaining at this point?

4. What diagnostic testing would you consider?

Cervical spine x-rays are unremarkable. NP testing reveals an elevated level of anxiety. Cognitive deficits are noted primarily related to attention and concentration.

5. What is your initial treatment plan for headaches and the cognitive deficits? If the initial plan is not successful, what might be appropriate next steps?

As part of the treatment plan, you suggest a referral to the Office of Vocational Rehabilitation to obtain support for return-to-work efforts. The patient says that her lawyer is not supportive of efforts to get her back to work.

6. How do you address this situation?

The patient wants you to say in your office note that all of her problems are a result of the crash and thinks you should not mention the preexisting anxiety.

7. How do you respond to this request?

Answers

1. Important details from the acute injury include a description of the accident, which can help with assessing initial injury severity. Initial treatment, such as whether the patient was taken immediately to the ED, and objective acute findings, such as the neurological examination in the ED and head CT findings will also be useful. A history of prior concussions and preexisting conditions such as migraine headaches or psychological difficulties is also useful as they may suggest a more prolonged recovery course. Active litigation may also be associated with more and more prolonged symptoms. Try to characterize the headaches based on presentation and also clarify examples of memory deficits. Assess for ongoing psychosocial stressors and behavioral changes. Ask about prior treatment for this injury and what interventions were and were not helpful.

2. The examination would to some degree be tailored to presenting symptoms. In this case, look for findings that may lead to or worsen headaches. Consider a detailed evaluation of eye function, and examine the neck and related structures for a cervicogenic component. Assess for temporomandibular dysfunction and neuralgia. Cognitively, evaluate short-term memory, attention, and concentration. Consider a validated cognitive test such as the MoCA. Also consider a test that assesses effort, such as the Rey 15-item test.

3. The patient appears to have posttraumatic headaches given her report of not having headaches before the crash. Further evaluation may lead to diagnosis of postconcussion disorder.

4. At this point, NP testing may be helpful. It can more clearly and objectively identify cognitive deficits, and the pattern of deficits may help clarify whether they are related to the crash or not. NP testing can also provide information regarding personality characteristics that may suggest a longer recovery period. Embedded measures of effort will be useful to help interpret results. Cervical x-rays could be considered.

5. The headaches appear to be primarily tension-type with a cervicogenic component. PT and nonsteroidal anti-inflammatory medications can be initiated. One should evaluate for causes of tension or cervical strain and intervene as appropriate. For the cognitive deficits, consider underlying reasons for decreased concentration and attention. Anxiety and poor sleep should be addressed. Psychological support/behavioral therapy may address both of these problems, but pharmacological intervention for sleep or anxiety can also be considered. Improvement in headache management may also help alleviate these cognitive problems. A course of cognitive therapy may also be beneficial. Ideally this would focus on specific problem areas that the patient identifies; for example, tasks at work. If deficits persist, pharmacological management—for example, a stimulant medication—could be considered.

6. It is possible that she would get a bigger settlement if she is deemed permanently unable to return to work. However, if she does have the potential to return to gainful employment, it is not likely that she will be able to hide this. In the long run, she may be better off psychologically and financially putting her efforts toward improvement (including vocational activity) rather than reinforcing her degree of disability. Ultimately, the patient must make the decision, but the physician should provide appropriate options and highlight potential benefits of returning to work. The patient can be reminded that the attorney can provide advice but that ultimately she needs to decide what is best for her.

7. You can tell the patient that it is not ethical to hide information. You can reassure her that you are comfortable pointing out in your report that the crash led to many of the problems that she is dealing with. You can also say that getting better is about more than just getting more money in a settlement and that there is no guarantee of a large monetary reward. Suggest to her that improving control of anxiety may make her life much better over a long period of time.

BIBLIOGRAPHY

Hanks RA, Rapport LJ, Seagly K, et al. Outcomes after concussion recovery education: effects of litigation and disability status on maintenance of symptoms. *J Neurotrauma*. 2019;36(4):554–558. https://doi.org/10.1089/neu.2018.5873

Iverson GL, Lange RT, Gaetz MB, et al. Mild traumatic brain injury. In: Zasler ND, et al., eds. *Brain Injury Medicine*. 2nd ed. Demos Medical; 2013:chap 29.

Watanabe TK. Post-traumatic headache. In: Zollman FS, ed. *Manual of Traumatic Brain Injury: Assessment and Management*. Demos Medical; 2016:chap 57.

A 23-year-old male is admitted to the inpatient brain injury rehabilitation unit after sustaining a TBI due to a high-speed motor vehicle crash 2 weeks ago. He is described as agitated. Staff are asking that you start some medications to help this problem.

Questions

1. What more do you need to know about his presentation in regard to these behavioral problems?

2. What would you look for when doing an examination?

He had no premorbid history of behavioral problems. He had bilateral fronto-temporal intracerebral hemorrhages on his head CT at the time of his injury. He has no known history of psychiatric problems or substance abuse. The initial medical workup does not reveal evidence of infection or electrolyte abnormalities. Sleep has been poor. He is disoriented. He is restless and yells but does not engage in conversation.

3. What causes for the agitation should be considered?

4. What tests or assessment tools may be ordered?

A CT scan does not demonstrate any new findings. An EEG cannot be obtained successfully due to the problematic behaviors. The Agitated Behavior Scale (ABS) demonstrates scores typically in the 30s (which is high) with scores highest for behaviors including impatience, resistance to care, pulling at tubes, and quick changes of mood. Sleep is decreased and fragmented.

5. What is an appropriate treatment plan at this point? How should this plan be modified if it is not helpful?

A nursing assistant comes to you extremely angry. She says the patient became sexually aggressive with her, exposing himself and using profane language. She no longer wants to care for the patient.

6. How can you help defuse the situation?

A family member calls, complaining that her loved one is being "drugged up."

7. How can you approach this person to provide a better understanding of the use of medications?

Answers

1. More details regarding the agitation are needed. The term "agitation" is not descriptive enough and people use it to describe many different behaviors. Nursing and therapy staff should be interviewed to characterize the problematic behaviors and determine triggers and their severity. Is the patient at risk of harming himself or others? Some behaviors may not require intervention. One must assess for comorbidities such as infections, metabolic disorders, hypoxia, electrolyte abnormalities, sleep deficits, painful conditions, or seizures that may be the cause of or contribute to the problem. Location of injury may be helpful; agitation is most frequently associated with orbitofrontal injuries. One would want to know if he had any premorbid behavioral issues or psychiatric disorders. Perhaps the problems are not completely new and have responded to certain medications in the past.

2. It will be helpful to determine his overall level of cognition. Assess memory, insight, and communicative ability. Look for painful conditions. Observe the problematic behaviors and attempts at interventions that may help or exacerbate the situation.

3. This behavior could be a direct manifestation of the brain trauma, especially given the frontotemporal injuries. Poor sleep can be exacerbating the problem. Medications should be reviewed as some can impact cognition or have direct adverse effects on behavior. Confusion and inability to communicate wants and needs can lead to agitated behavior. He may be exposed to overly stimulating environments.

4. If the agitation is a problem that has arisen after the prior CT report, further cerebral imaging may be useful to rule out a new central process. An EEG can rule out seizures as a cause. An objective measure of agitation, such as the ABS, can help to characterize the problematic behaviors and measure the effectiveness of the intervention plan implemented. A sleep log may help track sleep more objectively.

5. Consider pharmacological and nonpharmacological interventions to help with sleep. Continue to track this objectively. Avoid overstimulation (e.g., crowded rooms or television) and provide day/night cues, orientation cues, and quiet at night. Minimize and routinize patient care interactions. Ask the team to identify and track possible antecedents to the problematic behaviors. Consider initiation of a medication as a standing dose rather than PRN. It is often difficult to assess efficacy of PRN medications, as problematic behaviors are often at least somewhat self-limited. Mood-stabilizing medications such as valproic acid or carbamazepine can be considered. Antipsychotics and beta-blockers are other options, as are serotonergic medications. Be mindful of potential side effects of these medications. Assess efficacy using a validated outcome measure or by objectively assessing the quality and quantity of the specific targeted problematic behaviors. If the initial

medication does not work, consider changing dose or trying a different one. Reevaluate for medical complications. Reassess for possible undiagnosed painful conditions.

6. Staff on a brain injury unit should be trained about common behavioral problems in this population and have a basic understanding of why they occur. Sexually aggressive behavior should be treated by establishing firm limits, without escalating emotional responses. The psychologist may help develop cognitive behavioral approaches, including appropriate rewards and punishments to suppress these behaviors. Staff should also be supported.

7. It may be helpful to explain that medications can make the environment safer for the patient. Also, medications may help prevent the patient from hurting staff when they are performing needed care. Medications may prevent the need for restraints, which can be uncomfortable or cause injury. Let the family know that agitation is often a phase in brain injury recovery and that you will try to decrease medications as soon as possible once they are not needed. You can also assure them that you are constantly monitoring for possible side effects of medications.

BIBLIOGRAPHY

McAllister TW. Emotional and behavioral sequelae of traumatic brain injury. In: Zasler ND, et al., eds. *Brain Injury Medicine*. 2nd ed. Demos Medical; 2013:chap 62.

Williamson D, Frenette AJ, Burry LD, et al. Pharmacological interventions for agitated behaviours in patients with traumatic brain injury: a systematic review. *BMJ Open*. 2019;9(7):e029604. https://doi.org/10.1136/bmjopen-2019-029604

Yudolfsky SC, Silver JM, Anderson KE. Aggressive disorders. In: Arcineigas DB, Zasler ND, Vanderplog RD, Jaffee MS, eds. *Management of Adults with Traumatic Brain Injury*. American Psychiatric Association; 2013:chap 10.

A 45-year-old college professor fell down a flight of stairs when leaving the lecture hall and sustained a TBI. He was admitted to a hospital and was discharged after 2 days. You see him in the Physical Medicine and Rehabilitation (PM&R) outpatient clinic 2 weeks later for an initial evaluation for any sequelae from this injury.

Questions

1. What questions should you ask him to determine if he is having ongoing disability from this injury?

2. What elements of the physical examination would you be especially interested in performing?

You find that the head CT done in the hospital did not demonstrate any acute findings. On history-taking, he notes that he has difficulty concentrating and staying on task, and is easily distracted. He expresses distress regarding these problems. He denies vertigo, focal weakness, and balance or coordination problems, and has no headache or visual complaints. His Mini-Mental State Exam (MMSE) score is 30/30. He reports slight overall improvement since his injury and states that no new problems since then. No deficits are noted on cranial nerve examination, and strength, sensation, and balance are within normal limits. He appears somewhat anxious and verbose but can provide clear and accurate information regarding his injury course. He is significantly overweight.

3. What further problems should be considered that may be exacerbating these complaints?

4. What further diagnostic testing should or should not be considered at this time?

Upon further questioning, he reports preinjury difficulties with always feeling tired despite generally getting 7 to 8 hours of sleep at night. He uses diphenhydramine two to three times a week to help him sleep. Fatigue is a significant problem with his daily functioning. He says that he has a strong marriage but has been "in a bit of a funk" over the past couple of months since his mother passed away. He is feeling some pressure to return to work.

5. What is an appropriate treatment plan at this time? If problems do not resolve, what changes in management could be considered?

Six months later, he has still not successfully transitioned to his prior full academic teaching load. He recently had an independent medical examination that stated that based on the history, neurological examination, and the duration of time since injury, he was fully recovered and should be working full time.

6. How can you support the patient's contention that the injury has prevented him from returning to full-time work?

The speech therapist (a recent graduate) working with him complains that the patient is always "talking down to her" and saying that the activities that they work on are not worthwhile. She suggests that he does not respect women as much as men and wants the case reassigned to someone else.

7. How can you resolve this conflict?

Answers

1. One should ask about any problems that he has noticed. Ask about vocational and avocational activities, including both the quality and efficiency in performing tasks. Also ask about any changes in interactions with others. You may need to ask about difficulties with memory, attention, emotional lability, mood, headaches, vision, balance, and coordination. Some patients do not know that certain problems may be related to the brain injury and may not mention them without specifically asking about them.

2. The MMSE and MoCA are simple cognitive screening tools that can be done in the office but are not very sensitive. A standard neurologic exam including cranial nerves, finger-nose-finger, balance, and gait evaluation should be performed. Look for asymmetries in the motor, sensory, or reflex examination. A musculoskeletal screen for other possibly missed injuries should be completed.

3. Poor sleep, certain medications, anxiety, and depression can contribute to cognitive dysfunction. Psychosocial stressors may also be playing a role. Some of these issues may be premorbid but not evident regarding functional performance until now.

4. In the absence of new neurological findings and nonfocal examination, there is no need for further cerebral imaging at this time. It is too early to perform full NP testing, and there is limited utility for the briefer computerized cognitive testing in the absence of preinjury data. Evaluation of possible premorbid conditions that may exacerbate problems could be considered (e.g., sleep apnea).

5. As this is a relatively recent injury, it is appropriate to reassure him that he should continue to improve significantly. He should not over-exert himself physically or cognitively although a moderate degree of activity may be beneficial. Minimize medications that may have cognitive side effects, such as diphenhydramine. Cognitive rehabilitation should be prescribed, with a focus on return to work. To decrease stress, you can reassure him that he should not feel the need to return work before he is ready and that you can help provide his employer with the documentation needed to support this. When he does resume working, it will be helpful to ensure that he is performing well. Information regarding this may come from the patient, coworkers, and, in this case, perhaps student evaluations. If problems with fatigue persist, a workup for medical conditions (e.g., sleep apnea, endocrinopathies) can be considered. Given his premorbid difficulties, a formal sleep study may be useful. Sleep hygiene principles should be reviewed. Psychological support for his recent loss, adjustment to disability, and stress may also be helpful. Pharmacological intervention with an antidepressant may also be considered. If he is not fully recovered functionally within a few months, formal NP testing can be considered. If treatable medical causes for fatigue have been ruled out, a trial of a medication to help improve daytime alertness may be appropriate.

6. It is often argued that cognitive deficits after mild injuries should resolve quickly, usually within a few months. However, ongoing problems that may have been triggered or exacerbated by the TBI may affect cognitive and overall function, such as poor sleep, stress, or persistent headaches. It is therefore reasonable in this case to attribute his inability to achieve full-time employment to the injury.

7. It may be beneficial to suggest to the therapist that the patient may be defensive regarding the cognitive problems that are being pointed out, especially in this case where intellectual ability is so important, at least vocationally. Patients often have difficulty understanding that cognitive skills worked on in therapy may be generalizable to other activities that the patient may see as more relevant. You may suggest that the speech therapist work with the patient on activities that are more clearly related to what the patient sees as valuable; for example, teaching. It may also be helpful to reinforce with the patient the rationale for cognitive therapy and its importance in getting allowing him to achieve his goal for successful return to work.

BIBLIOGRAPHY

Ciccerone, KD. Cognitive rehabilitation. In: Zasler ND, et al., eds. *Brain Injury Medicine*. 2nd ed. Demos Medical; 2013:chap 61.

Cicerone KD, Goldin E, Ganci K, et al. Evidence-based cognitive rehabilitation: systematic review of the literature from 2009 through 2014. *Arch Phys Med Rehabil*. 2019;100(8):1515–1533. https://doi.org/10.1016/j.apmr.2019.02.011

Cronin H, O'Loughlin E. Sleep and fatigue after TBI. *NeuroRehabilitation*. 2018;43(3):307–317. https://doi.org/10.3233/NRE-182484

A 65-year-old woman is seen in your clinic. She has a family history of idiopathic Parkinson's disease (PD), and she is concerned she is developing symptoms.

Questions

1. What more do you want to know about the patient's history, comorbidities, and social situation? Please tell me why you are asking for these specifics.

2. How would you go about performing a physical exam on this patient? Why are these maneuvers/exam components important?

She has not been on any neuroleptic medications but was started on amiodarone recently for arrhythmia. The patient shows signs of hypo- and bradykinesia with masked face and a resting tremor that affects the right arm more than the left. She has noticed a gradual onset of symptoms over the last 12 months.

3. What is the differential diagnosis for this patient? Tell me the most likely diagnosis and why it is the most likely.

4. What diagnostic test or tests would you order and why?

Functional imaging (DaTscan) is unavailable. MRI is normal. CSF analysis is unavailable.

5. Outline the treatment plan. Please tell me about the initial treatment and next steps if that fails.

Your patient is diagnosed with PD. Her mother died after a prolonged course of PD with poor quality of life at the end of her life. She would like to be reassured that if/when her mental condition deteriorates, she does not go through what her mother did.

6. How would you facilitate her care and her wishes?

You suggest a course of rehabilitation with PT, OT, and speech therapies. Your patient confronts you angrily by saying "I have a degenerative condition. What is therapy going to do for me?"

7. Tell me in lay terms about the role of rehabilitation in PD.

Answers

1. Demographics are important, as PD is less common in African Americans and Asians. Where the patient lives and grew up is important because there is increased risk in rural areas, possibly due to exposure to pesticides. There is no evidence for trauma increasing the risk of PD. PD is twice as common in men as in women. Family history can increase risk, although only 5% to 10% of all cases are genetic in nature. Family history for other neurodegenerative diseases (i.e., progressive supranuclear palsy) should be obtained as they can sometimes be mistaken for PD. The examiner should inquire about hypo- and bradykinesia, resting tremor, postural instability, and rigidity, as these are the cardinal features of PD. The examiner should ask about exposure to medications including neuroleptics, metoclopramide, lithium, and amiodarone, as these can cause symptoms of parkinsonism. History of TBI, stroke, brain tumor, and metabolic encephalopathy should also be obtained as consequences of these conditions can also mimic PD.

2. Observe for resting tremor, particularly in the hand. Pill-rolling tremor is seen in 50% of patients. The tremor is observed when the hand is motionless but abolishes with complete relaxation or with voluntary movement. Rigidity is present with passive range of motion as a resistance that is present evenly throughout the entire range. Hypokinesia is manifested by decreased blink rate and decreased facial movement that causes an expressionless "masked" appearance, and overall fewer small shifts of position. Other elements of hypo- and bradykinesia include micrographia and softened and monotonous speech. Ambulation should be examined for signs of shuffling and festination (short rapid steps to avoid falling). Postural instability is manifested as impaired righting reactions to postural perturbations. She has no cognitive symptoms.

3. The differential diagnosis for this patient involves conditions that cause parkinsonism, degenerative diseases, and diseases that cause tremor. Medication exposure to neuroleptics, metoclopramide, lithium, and amiodarone can cause parkinsonism. Normal pressure hydrocephalus, progressive supranuclear palsy, TBI, brain tumor, paraneoplastic illness, and metabolic or viral encephalopathy can also mimic PD symptoms. Essential tremor is more likely to be present with volitional movements than the resting tremor of PD. The most likely diagnosis in this patient is idiopathic PD. Early PD is most often characterized by hypo- and bradykinesia and tremor. Parkinsonism caused by medication is more likely to present as rapid onset.

4. PD diagnosis is largely based on clinical exam and history. The diagnosis should involve serial examination over time and trial of dopaminergic medication. Functional imaging can be considered in early cases or in cases that are ambiguous. 123I-ioflupane single-photon emission computerized tomography (SPECT) imaging (also known as DaTscan), F-DOPA PET scan, and FP-CIT are examples of functional imaging tests evaluating dopamine

activity in the brain. Standard MRI has little utility. There are no clinically useful CSF-based tests.

5. The mainstays of PD diagnosis remain the clinical exam and history, as well as a trial with a dopaminergic medication. The patient should be examined repeatedly over time to monitor for new symptoms and/or progression of symptoms that can make the diagnosis clearer. Additionally, a trial with a dopaminergic medication is warranted. The symptoms of idiopathic PD respond to a trial of levodopa-carbidopa or a dopamine agonist much more reliably than the other conditions on the differential diagnosis list. If this fails, consider functional imaging.

6. The risk of dementia is increased with PD. An estimated 10% to 15% of patients with PD will go on to develop dementia. Your patient should be counseled about writing a living will or preparing advanced directives. She should identify a person to be her durable power of attorney should she become mentally incapacitated. She should make sure that person knows her wishes not only about resuscitation, but also mechanical ventilation, enteral nutrition, life-prolonging medications, dialysis, and rehospitalizations.

7. Rehabilitation can be effective in the short term in improving quality of walking, activities of daily living (getting dressed/washed, toileting), speech quality, and cognition. Therapies can also be helpful for providing adaptive equipment and improving home safety. Gains made in rehabilitation are lost over time due to the degenerative nature of the disease. For this reason, patients should be sent to PT, OT, and speech therapy every 6 to 12 months.

BIBLIOGRAPHY

Radhakrishnan DM, Goyal V. Parkinson's disease: a review. *Neurol India* [serial online]. 2018 [cited 2020 Aug 26];66(Suppl S1):26–35. https://doi.org/10.4103/0028-3886.226451

Ropper AH, Samuels MA, Klein JP, et al., eds. *Adams and Victor's Principles of Neurology, 11e.* McGraw-Hill: Degenerative diseases of the nervous system; August 25, 2020:chap 38.

Saulino M, Doherty J, Fried G. Rehabilitation concerns in degenerative movement disorders of the central nervous system. In: Braddom RL, ed. *Physical Medicine and Rehabilitation.* 3rd ed. Saunders; 2007:chap 52.

CASE 9

The patient is a 65-year-old male with a history of hypertension who was brought to the hospital 1 week ago after experiencing a generalized tonic-clonic seizure. Initial imaging showed a right frontal mass with surrounding edema. He was brought to the OR for R frontal craniotomy and resection of the tumor. He has been extubated and is tolerating an oral diet. The acute care team feels that he is stable and ready for discharge.

Questions

1. What more do you want to know about the patient's history, present status, and social situation? Please tell me why you are asking for these specifics.

2. How would you go about performing a physical exam on this patient? Why are these maneuvers/exam components important?

The patient is able to share with you that he is a practicing attorney and this seizure occurred at the office last week while he was working on an important case. He is eager to return to work and get back to this case. He does drive an automobile and he displays poor insight into his condition and reasons why he may not be able to return to work or driving right away. He is divorced and lives alone. He has three adult children who live relatively close by. His home is a two-story home with three steps to enter, with the bedroom and bathrooms upstairs. His physical exam is notable for a flat affect, left-sided weakness with normal to low muscle tone. His immediate and delayed recall were 3/3, but he needed one semantic cue for delayed recall. His abstract reasoning and problem-solving are moderately impaired. He has been seen by PT and they have documented that he is able to ambulate 50 feet with a walker and minimal assistance. His pathology results are pending and his team reports that he can follow up with neuro-oncology and radiation oncology "after rehab" to discuss his treatment plan. Current medications include levetiracetam, dexamethasone, and quetiapine. You plan to refer him to acute inpatient rehabilitation.

3. What are some questions that you might have for his current team regarding his medications?

4. What additional diagnostic testing are you interested in tracking down before you formulate your rehabilitation plan?

Postoperative MRI showed a total resection of the tumor. Pathology is consistent glioblastoma multiforme. The neurosurgery team indicates that levetiracetam and dexamethasone will be tapered off. Quetiapine had been started for agitation. The patient's children are distraught. They want to know why you are recommending rehabilitation and not hospice.

5. Outline the treatment plan. How do you explain your rationale for inpatient rehabilitation?

The patient has progressed well in inpatient rehabilitation, and he is ready for discharge. He will be going home, with one of his children staying with him initially to provide some supervision and assistance. The patient wants to know how he can continue to work toward the goal of returning to work.

6. How care might his outpatient care be facilitated? How will you handle his request to work on going back to work?

Over the next few months, the patient is able to successfully return to work and drive a car. He develops some fatigue and finds that he is not able to tolerate a full workday without some rest breaks. You provide a prescription for methylphenidate, which is helpful. Fortunately, his law practice also is very accommodating, and with the accommodations, he is happy and satisfied that he is able to continue to maintain his career. He comes to the office with his daughter, who is very upset with you for allowing him to continue to exert himself by working full time. In her view, the exertion of working full time is placing him at risk for a more rapid decline. She confronts you at the visit and wants you to persuade him to retire.

7. How would you resolve this conflict?

Answers

1. It is important to have a picture of his prior functional status, including his functional mobility and self-care. This will have implications not only for his short-term rehabilitation goals and prognosis for post-op functional recovery, but also his prognosis overall. You will also want to know if he was working and if he was a driver. It is also important to ascertain his social history in terms of household/family members available to provide care and/or support. He may need physical and/or cognitive support once he goes home. You will also need to know about any architectural barriers in the home. You will also want to have a discussion with his team about what his treatment plan might be. Are they planning chemotherapy, radiation? What is the timeline for these interventions? You will want to know if he has any complaints of pain or headache at this time, as these may impact him functionally. Finally, you want to know what he is currently able to do functionally. Has he been out of bed? Have PT/OT and speech therapy seen the patient? Does he have dysphagia? Finally, you want to be sure to ask the patient about his mood and how he is responding emotionally to all that is happening.

2. The physical exam would be comprised of a general neurologic exam. This should include level of arousal, orientation, cranial nerves, and language and motor function including tone, power, and coordination. You will want to do some baseline cognitive screening to get an idea of any cognitive deficits. This can include immediate and delayed recall (I will give you three things to remember, you can repeat them now and I will ask you to recall them in five minutes), serial sevens, or simple mental calculation such as adding coins. You will want to take note of the patient's affect and amount of psychomotor activity. It is also helpful to ask conversational style questions to evaluate his insight into his condition and his judgment as well as his capacity for problem-solving.

3. Since routine prophylactic use of anticonvulsants is not recommended beyond the immediate postoperative period, particularly in patients who are medically stable, you will want to inquire if there is a plan to taper his levetiracetam since that is a medication that may have cognitive side effects. Similarly, you will want to ask why the patient has been started on quetiapine so that you can plan to wean it if possible. You will want to know what the plan is for dexamethasone. Is it being tapered? Has he had any problems with steroid-induced hyperglycemia?

4. You will want to know if postoperative MRI showed a total or near-total resection of his tumor as this will confer a better prognosis. You will want to know the pathology of the tumor.

5. Admit the patient to inpatient rehabilitation. A social worker will need to assist the team in providing the patient and family support through the rehabilitation process and also to help formulate a safe discharge plan. The social worker

will likely also need to help the patient and family identify caregivers to provide physical and/or cognitive assistance after discharge from inpatient rehab. PT will need to work with him to achieve safe functional mobility within the home, including negotiation of stairs. They will also help, along with occupational and speech therapists, determine the level of care needed upon discharge, and provide family/caregiver education and instruction. OT will be important for similarly addressing self-care but also for ongoing surveillance of the patient's cognitive recovery along with speech therapy. Speech therapy will evaluate for cognitive linguistic deficits and help the team and the physiatrist place these deficits into the greater context of the patient's current recovery and goals for beyond discharge such as return to work. The speech language pathologist will also need to evaluate for potential dysphagia and treat accordingly. The patient has several circumstances which confer a more favorable prognosis. Factors indicating a more favorable prognosis include initial presentation of seizure, tumor location in the frontal lobe, high functional status, and complete surgical resection. You can share with the family that the patient may eventually be hospice appropriate if he experiences tumor recurrences and is not deemed a candidate for surgery or chemotherapy or experiences a significant decline in functional status or neurologic status despite treatment. You emphasize that at this juncture, the benefits of inpatient rehabilitation are well documented and that there is a favorable prognosis for a more immediate improvement in his level of function and quality of life.

6. The first step after discharge home will be to refer to outpatient therapies to continue to maximize functional independence. You should explain that his outpatient speech and occupational therapists can challenge him more in terms of work-specific tasks. At that point, it may be beneficial to involve a neuropsychologist to evaluate cognitive strengths and weaknesses and recommend individualized strategies to maximize the chances of successful work reentry. It is important to have a frank discussion about the nature of his illness and the impact that his future treatments may have on his level of function. He may experience headaches, fatigue, and decreased activity tolerance. He may experience recurrence or other complications of treatment that also impact his function. You can explain that you can continue to work with him throughout his course to help optimize his function and quality of life at every stage.

7. You are ethically bound by the principles of respect for your patient's autonomy and respect for his personhood. Although you cannot concede to her request and recommend her father stop working, you should show empathy for her and recognize that she is trying to cope with her father's terminal illness. You can share that he is happy and fulfilled by working at the present time and he has progressed well through the rehabilitation process and has demonstrated that he can tolerate his present activity pattern. You can promise them both that you will continue to follow him as a patient and modify your recommendations and treatment as things change.

BIBLIOGRAPHY

Ricard D, Idbaih A, Ducray F, et al. Primary brain tumours in adults. *Lancet.* 2012;379(9830):1984–1996. https://doi.org/10.1016/S0140-6736(11)61346-9

Thakkar P, Greenwald BD, Patel P. Rehabilitation of adult patients with primary brain tumors: a narrative review. *Brain Sci.* 2020;10:492. https://doi.org/10.3390/brainsci10080492

A 27-year-old woman has had multiple sclerosis (MS) for 5 years. She is finding it more difficult to walk recently over the summer. She is on a beta-interferon but takes no other medications. Her last acute flare was 2 years ago. Vitals are normal.

Questions

1. What are the key elements that you would like to obtain regarding this patient's history and review of systems? Explain why these elements are important.

She tells you that this has been a gradual insidious worsening, mainly due to stiffness in her legs. She also fatigues easily. She also admits to some depressed mood.

2. What is critical to do on physical exam?

Her mental status, cranial nerves, sensation, and coordination are intact. Strength is 5/5, but she has modified Ashworth scale 2 tone in her lower limbs, especially adductors, ankle plantar flexion, and inversion. She has three beats of clonus in both ankles. Her gait is a spastic diplegic pattern. Range of motion at hips, knees, and ankles is full. Skin is intact.

3. What is the differential diagnosis of her difficulty walking? What diagnostic testing, if any, is indicated?

MRI shows plaques in the thoracic cord and periventricular white matter, which are unchanged from 2 years ago. Urinalysis is normal. Her Patient Health Questionnaire (PHQ)-9 score indicates moderate depression severity?

4. What interventions would help her improve her function and quality of life?

She works as an elementary school teacher but is finding it difficult to continue working. She wants to apply for Social Security.

5. What advice would you give her regarding applying for Social Security?

You recommend an ankle-foot orthosis, but the patient is reluctant to use this because of cosmesis.

6. How would you try to convince her to use this device?

Answers

1. The course of her MS is critical to assess (relapse or insidious progression). This has important implications as far as her prognosis and will guide the physiatrist in plotting her rehabilitation course. It is also important to ask for more details regarding the onset of her ambulatory difficulties. Did it come about gradually or suddenly? Was there a precipitant in the form of an infection or injury? What is her typical activity pattern? Screening her for depression is also vitally important, as depression significantly impacts quality of life. This can be done with a depression screening tool such as the PHQ-9, which is a validated depression screening tool. Review of symptoms should include vision changes, tremor, fatigue, heat sensitivity, weakness in limbs, spasms, and bladder changes.

2. Physical exam includes cranial nerves, sensation, coordination, strength, muscle tone, reflexes, range of motion, and gait analysis.

3. As far as differential diagnosis, this patient may be experiencing an MS flare, secondary progressive disease, a "pseudo-flare" from infection or other stressor, heat sensitivity, ataxia, or the effects of spasticity. Tests: MRI, urinalysis.

4. Treatment includes multidisciplinary rehabilitation including PT for gait training and stretching, maintaining cool environment, orthotics prescription, spasticity management, and dalfampridine (Ampyra). Corticosteroids or adrenocorticotropic hormone (ACTH) and plasmapheresis are not indicated as this is secondary progressive MS and not a flare. For depression, she should be referred for cognitive behavioral therapy (CBT).

5. Social Security requires documentation of total and permanent disability (inability to perform any kind of work for which she is educationally qualified). Discuss reasonable accommodation under the Americans with Disability Act (e.g., air conditioning, teaching while seated, teacher's aide, first floor classroom).

6. Be empathetic and acknowledge her concerns. "I understand that you might be a little turned off by the appearance of a brace. Let's talk about that." You can discuss how an ankle-foot orthosis (AFO) can give one a more normal-appearing gait pattern, decrease her risk of falling, and decrease the energy of gait so she can feel less tired. You should also discuss how a molded AFO can be hidden by slacks.

BIBLIOGRAPHY

Khan F, Amatya B. Rehabilitation in multiple sclerosis: a systematic review of systematic reviews. *Arch Phys Med Rehabil.* 2017;98(2):353–367. https://doi.org/10.1016/j.apmr.2016.04.016

Kroenke K, Spitzer RL, Williams JB. The PHQ-9: validity of a brief depression severity measure. *J Gen Intern Med.* 2001;16(9):606–613. https://doi.org/10.1046/j.1525-1497.2001.016009606.x

Samkoff LM, Goodman AD. Symptomatic management in multiple sclerosis. *Neurol Clin.* 2011;29(2):449–463. https://doi.org/10.1016/j.ncl.2011.01.008

Shah A, Flores A, Nourbaksh B, et al. Multiple sclerosis. In: Cifu DX, ed. *Braddom's Physical Medicine and Rehabilitation.* 5th ed. Elsevier; 2015: 1029–1052.

3 Cancer and Other Medically Related Impairments

Julie K. Silver

A 70-year-old man presents to your cancer rehabilitation program with recently diagnosed oropharyngeal cancer. He is starting chemoradiation therapy and will undergo a right-sided modified radical neck dissection in a few weeks.

Questions

1. What additional history would you like to know?

2. What should you focus on with your physical exam?

He describes some fatigue related to the antineoplastic treatment, and on physical examination, he has some baseline mild loss of cervical range of motion, particularly in bilateral lateral rotation. He has mild chronic obstructive pulmonary disease and uses an inhaler infrequently. He quit smoking 2 years ago. You have sent him for a prehabilitation program focusing on prevention of common complications.

3. What complications would you be concerned about?

He returns to your clinic 3 months after surgery. He has had the surgery and is aphonic. He reports neck and right shoulder pain.

4. What is the differential diagnosis for these complaints, and what physical exam findings and diagnostic tests would help establish a diagnosis?

He has normal shoulder range of motion with a negative impingement sign. He has right inferolateral scapular winging with shoulder shrug. Electromyography (EMG) shows positive sharp waves and large amplitude motor unit potentials (MUPs) with decreased recruitment in the trapezius.

5. What is the diagnosis and how would you treat this condition?

You are interested in seeing more patients like this and expanding your head and neck cancer rehabilitation program.

6. How would you go about this?

He undergoes video-fluoroscopy swallow evaluation, which demonstrates aspiration of all consistencies of liquids and solids. The speech-language pathologist recommends that he be NPO (nothing by mouth) and should have a percutaneous endoscopically placed gastrostomy (PEG) tube. He refuses, saying food is his only joy.

7. How should you respond?

Answers

1. You would want to know his goals. What are his current symptoms? You ask about comorbidities. You ask if he has any side effects from his chemoradiation therapy, especially numbness, fatigue, and pain.

2. You would want to examine his neck for lymphadenopathy and determine range of motion of his neck and shoulders. A careful neurologic exam should include a thorough examination for cranial nerve and sensory deficits.

3. Common complications from treatment of head and neck cancers include cosmetic deformity, dysphagia, pain in neck and shoulders, nerve damage to spinal accessory nerve and brachial plexus, fatigue, and depression.

4. The differential diagnoses include rotator cuff impingement, radiation fibrosis, spinal accessory palsy, lymphedema, and/or brachial plexopathy. Physical exam should include range of motion, palpation for lymphedema, and observation of scapular motion during shoulder flexion and shrugging. Electrodiagnostic testing will be useful.

5. The likely diagnosis is spinal accessory nerve palsy. Physical therapy, including taping, and neuromuscular stimulation may help. Gabapentin, pregabalin, and/or selective serotonin-norepinephrine reuptake inhibitors (SSNRIs) may help with neuropathic pain. A tricyclic antidepressant medication should probably not be used in an older man, especially if he has benign prostatic hypertrophy, due to the risk of urinary retention. These medications are similar to what would be considered first-line treatment for chemotherapy-induced peripheral neuropathy as well.

6. One should be empathetic and listen to his concerns. He is an adult and has every right to refuse the procedure. After listening, remind him that nutrition is critical to his quality of life. The enteral feedings may well be temporary until he regains strength in his pharyngeal muscles. Express your concern regarding his ability to maintain his nutrition without getting aspiration-related pneumonia. He can then make an informed decision.

7. Marketing the program should be targeted at the treating physicians such as otolaryngologists, head and neck cancer surgeons, and medical and radiation oncologists. In addition, nurse navigators, nurse practitioners, and/or physician assistants are often the primary referring providers for these services. Attending tumor boards or cancer committee meetings help facilitate these connections.

BIBLIOGRAPHY

Bulsara VM, Worthington HV, Glenny AM, et al. Interventions for the treatment of oral and oropharyngeal cancers: surgical treatment. *Cochrane Database Syst Rev.* December 24, 2018;12(12):CD006205. https://doi.org/10.1002/14651858. CD006205.pub4. PMID: 30582609; PMCID: PMC6517307.

Fradkin M, Batash R, Elmaleh S, et al. Management of peripheral neuropathy induced by chemotherapy. *Curr Med Chem.* 2019;26(25):4698–4708. https://doi.org/10.2174/0929867326666190107163756. PMID: 30621553.

A 60-year-old woman sees you for the first time and reports that 1 year ago she was diagnosed with breast cancer and underwent a right mastectomy with a sentinel lymph node biopsy followed by chemotherapy and radiation therapy. She reports that the reason she came to see you is that her right arm started swelling.

Questions

1. What are the most important questions in the history to help sort out the etiology?

2. What are important aspects of her physical exam?
She has painless swelling that developed gradually over the last 2 weeks.

Her last visit with oncology did not show any evidence of disease recurrence.

Her physical examination reveals mild swelling of the right arm and hand.

The extremity is soft to the touch and has pitting edema that is reversible.

There is a palpable cord in the axilla, but no breast masses or lymphadenopathy.

Stemmert sign is negative, and there is no bony tenderness.

3. What is the differential diagnosis of her arm swelling?

4. Which diagnostic tests are helpful for the arm swelling?

Her lymphoscintigraphy showed occlusion at the axilla. Doppler was negative.

5. What treatment would you recommend?

Her sleeve has worn out, and she says that she cannot afford a replacement garment, as her medical insurance will not cover this.

6. What approaches can you offer?

She returns 2 years later with exacerbation of her lymphedema. You note that she is not wearing her compression garments.

7. How would you approach this with her?

Answers

1. Is it painful? The hallmark of lymphedema is painless swelling, so if she says it hurts, then lymphedema is less likely than other conditions. You should also ask about fever, erythema, warmth, or drainage (for cellulitis). History of lymph node dissection or sentinel node biopsy makes lymphedema more likely. Late-stage cancer would trigger more concerns about metastasis. History of coagulopathy or atrial fibrillation might trigger thought for deep venous thrombosis.

2. Look for erythema. Palpate for lymphadenopathy and axillary cords. Examine both breasts for lumps. Check shoulder range of motion. Check for Stemmert sign (swelling in the web space of fingers or toes, which is consistent with lymphadenopathy and inconsistent with vascular edema or lipedema).

3. The differential diagnosis includes deep venous thrombosis, lipedema, and metastatic disease to bone. The most likely diagnosis is lymphedema.

4. A Doppler ultrasound to rule out deep venous thrombosis is warranted given the acute onset of swelling. Lymphoscintigraphy identifies abnormalities of the lymphatic system. If metastasis is suspected, particularly though not exclusively if her breast cancer was in a more advanced stage at diagnosis, a metastatic workup may be indicated. Physiatrists should work closely with oncologists when recommending a metastatic workup, regardless of who orders the imaging tests, as these often involve multimodal imaging with whole-body imaging techniques such as bone one scintigraphy, whole-body hybrid imaging (PET-CT and/or PET-MRI), or whole-body magnetic resonance imaging (WBMRI).

5. Treatment generally includes complete decongestive therapy (CDT) performed by a clinician with specialized training in lymphedema therapy. This consists of manual lymphatic drainage (MLD), which is decompressive manual therapy followed by application of compression tapes, and then prescription compression garments. Resistive weight training is indicated, not contraindicated, and can help improve function.

6. Compression garments are frequently not covered by insurance. Sometimes funding can be found through charitable organizations. You may have to compromise and go with a less expensive alternative like Ace wrapping.

7. Do not assume that her noncompliance is from a lack of motivation. Her compression garments may have worn out, and she might not have insurance coverage or funding to replace them. Perhaps she finds it difficult to wear them in hot weather. Ask the reasons and problem solve with her how to overcome them.

BIBLIOGRAPHY

Bagay L. Lymphedema. In: Frontera WR, Silver JK, Rizzo TD Jr, eds. *Essentials of Physical Medicine and Rehabilitation.* 4th ed. Elsevier; 2019:chap 132:735–739.

Pesapane F, Downey K, Rotili A, et al. Imaging diagnosis of metastatic breast cancer. *Insights Imaging.* June 16, 2020;11(1):79. https://doi.org/10.1186/s13244-020-00885-4. PMID: 32548731; PMCID: PMC7297923.

A 26-year-old man was diagnosed with acute myeloid leukemia. He comes to see you for fatigue and problems functioning in general.

Questions

1. What questions do you want to ask him about his cancer or his oncological treatment?

2. What is important to focus on in the physical exam?

You learn that he finished all of his treatment 3 months ago, and has no known active cancer in his body. He hopes that he is cured. He received cytarabine and daunomycin. On review of systems, he tells you that he does not feel refreshed after sleep. He lost 30 pounds during treatment, but has gained 10 pounds back. He denies dyspnea, chest pain, or palpitations. He denies depression, and is optimistic about his recovery. His body mass index (BMI) is 20. Heart, lung, and motor exam is normal.

3. What is the differential diagnosis of his fatigue?

4. What diagnostic tests would be indicated?

His hemoglobin was 11.5. Prealbumin was within normal limits. Echocardiogram was normal.

5. Outline a treatment program.

He has missed substantial time from his work as a plumber. He is worried about losing his job.

6. What legal protections does he have?

7. Explain cancer-related fatigue to the patient in lay terms.

Answers

1. It is important to know if he is receiving active cancer treatment and what kind. It is also important to know if he has residual cancer and whether he is deemed curable. Ask about other medications he is taking. How is he sleeping? How is his mood? Does he have any dyspnea? How is his appetite, and has he lost weight?

2. Assess his BMI. Look for cachexia. Listen to his heart and lungs and assess his muscle strength.

3. Fatigue may be from insomnia, sleep apnea, side effects of medications, anemia, chronic infection, or cardiopulmonary or neuromuscular impairments. In particular, daunorubicin can cause cardiomyopathy, so this must be ruled out. Cancer-related fatigue is by definition a distressing and subjective sense of physical, emotional, and/or cognitive tiredness that is related to cancer or its treatment. Cancer-related fatigue is not proportional to one's activity level and often isn't responsive to rest or sleep.

4. A complete blood count (CBC) can rule out anemia and infection. Albumin or prealbumin levels can assess malnutrition. Echocardiogram can rule out cardiomyopathy.

5. Both cardiovascular and strength training exercises have been shown to reduce symptoms of cancer-related fatigue. Usually, modest exercise intensity levels (up to 60% of maximum oxygen consumption) for 5 days per week is tolerated by patients even if they are undergoing active cancer treatment. However, appropriate precautions and contraindications should always be adhered to with all patients, particularly those in active treatment.

6. The Family Medical Leave Act provides for up to 12 weeks per year of unpaid leave from work, prohibiting employers from terminating employees if they have a documented medical condition. Once he is ready to return to work, the Americans with Disabilities Act requires employers to make reasonable accommodations as long as the employee can perform the essential job requirements.

7. Cancer-related fatigue is a very common phenomenon impacting almost three-fourths of cancer patients. While it can be related to chemotherapy or radiation, it often persists long after treatment is completed. Patients feel tired despite getting adequate rest. There can be difficulty concentrating. Counterintuitively, the treatment is not rest but rather graded exercise.

BIBLIOGRAPHY

Cheville A. Cancer-related fatigue. In: Frontera WL, Silver JK, Rizzo TD Jr, eds. *Essentials of Physical Medicine and Rehabilitation.* 4th ed. Elsevier; 2019:chap 124:684–688.

Hussain Y, Miller S. Other myopathies. *Neurol Clin.* August 2020;38(3):619–635. https://doi.org/10.1016/j.ncl.2020.04.002. PMID: 32703473.

CASE 4

You are consulted on a 45-year-old who had a craniotomy for resection of a solitary right parietal brain tumor 4 days ago. The primary team would like to transfer him to inpatient rehabilitation.

Questions

1. What more do you want to know about the patient's history, comorbidities, and social situation? Please tell me why you are asking for these specifics.

2. How would you go about performing a physical exam on this patient? Why are these maneuvers/exam components important?

He presented to the hospital after a seizure, and MRI showed the brain mass. A workup with PET-CT, colonoscopy, and tumor markers failed to find a primary tumor, so he underwent resection. Frozen section consistent but not definitive for glioma. Pre-op he was independent and working as a middle school teacher. He now requires assistance with all mobility and self-care. He has a mild headache. He is incontinent of bowel and bladder. On exam he is alert, oriented with a mini-mental status of 25/30. His strength is 2/5 on the left. He has a left visual field cut and left hemi-neglect on double simultaneous tactile stimulation.

3. What is the differential diagnosis for this patient? Tell me the most likely diagnosis and why.

4. What further information do you need to know in order to determine what rehabilitation level of care is appropriate for him?

He is participating well with physical and occupational therapy. He lives in a one-story home with a three-step entry, with his wife who is also a school teacher. They have two teenage children at home. His spouse will take some time off work when he first comes home. No radiation or chemotherapy has yet been scheduled, as they are awaiting final tissue diagnosis. However, if it is glioblastoma multiforme, he will be recommended to receive temozolomide, an oral chemotherapy agent, and whole-brain radiation for 30 sessions, 5 days/week. Your rehabilitation unit is able to provide this during his rehabilitation. After discussion with the patient and his wife, he agrees to admission to the hospital inpatient rehabilitation unit.

5. Describe his rehab program.

You have recommended an inpatient rehab admission, but the insurance utilization reviewer denies coverage for the stay, stating, "why would we approve an expensive rehab program for someone with a terminal illness?"

6. How would you advocate for your patient?

You have won your appeal and he is admitted to your rehab unit. Four days into the stay, the final pathology is back, and it is glioblastoma multiforme. The neurosurgeon has just informed the patient of his diagnosis and prognosis. He is in tears when you walk into his room. "Why should I do all this when I'm going to die anyway?" he asks.

7. How would you approach this conversation?

Answers

1. Ask him about symptoms, including hemiparesis, sensation, vision, headaches, and spasms. Review the chart to see if pathology is back. Review the chart regarding whether he underwent a preoperative workup for metastatic disease. Ask him about his home setup and family support. What is his previous and current functional status? Ask him what he knows and wants to know about his diagnosis.

2. Review vitals. Listen to heart and lungs and check for calf edema or tenderness. Do a thorough neurologic exam including visual fields, strength sensation, and double simultaneous stimulation to look for hemi-neglect. Do a mental status exam.

3. This is most likely a primary brain tumor, and the most common (and worst prognosis) in adults is glioblastoma multiforme.

4. His goals are critical. Does he want to participate in an intensive rehab program in order to get home and is his home setup realistic? Can he tolerate ≥3 hours of therapy daily? Does he have upcoming chemotherapy and/or radiotherapy, and if so, can the rehabilitation program accommodate that?

5. His rehab will focus on practical skills for mobility and activities of daily living. His left neglect is likely to be a barrier and a major focus of therapy efforts. He will be on a dexamethasone taper and will need to be monitored for cerebral edema as well as steroid side effects including hyperglycemia, delirium, and myopathy.

6. First, ask for a peer-to-peer review, preferably with a physical medicine and rehabilitation (PM&R) physician. Present the goals for the admission. Present the literature that shows that brain tumor patients do as well in inpatient rehab as traumatic brain injury patients.

7. Ask the patient what he knows about his diagnosis, prognosis, and the efficacy of the proposed treatment. Ask what is important to him for his remaining life. Is being more functional, and less of a burden on his family, important to him? Offer consults to palliative care, psychology, and or pastoral care.

BIBLIOGRAPHY

Thakar P, Greenwald BD, Patel P. Rehabilitation of adult with primary brain tumors. *Brain Sci.* 2020;10(8):492–510. https://doi.org/10.3390/brainsci10080492

Vargo M. Brain tumor rehabilitation. *Am J Phys Med Rehabil.* 2011;90(5 suppl 1):S50–S62. https://doi.org/10.1097/PHM.0b013e31820be31f

4 Cardiovascular and Pulmonary Rehabilitation

Matthew N. Bartels

A 61-year-old man who was admitted with acute onset of substernal chest pain is seen in the ICU of the local hospital. He was admitted through the ED a day ago and underwent emergency surgery last night. He is now being evaluated after being stabilized for rehabilitation needs.

Questions

1. What more do you want to know about the patient's history, comorbidities, and social situation? Please tell me why you are asking for these specifics.

2. How would you go about performing a physical exam on this patient? Why are these maneuvers/exam components important?

You learn he had elevated troponin on admission with an EKG consistent with an anterior wall infarction. Cardiac catheterization was done, which showed four-vessel coronary disease with a left anterior descending coronary artery (LAD) occlusion that could not be opened via angioplasty. Subsequently, he had an emergent median sternotomy with coronary artery bypass graft x4. He had a cross-clamp time of 1 hour with a bypass time of 2.5 hours. When you see him in the ICU you were told he was very agitated earlier but is now calmer after being sedated. On your examination, he appears sleepy, but he is responsive to your stimulation. By report, he has had an otherwise relatively uncomplicated operative course. Asking him how he feels, you find that he has incisional pain, fatigue, mild shortness of breath, and loss of appetite. He has no focal neurologic complaints, but says: "I haven't really been awake long enough to check everything out yet." Exam shows a mild sternal click on cough, and he has palpable motion with movement. There are decreased breath sounds at the left lung base. He has a chest tube still in with no air leak and minimal drainage. There are transcutaneous pacing wires in place. There is mild erythema at the saphenous vein graft (SVG) donor sites but no clear infection, with soft calves and no edema. He has stable blood pressure and no orthostasis. His neurological exam appears fine as he has sensation and antigravity strength in arms and legs; he has no focal cranial nerve issues.

3. What is the differential diagnosis for this patient? Tell me the most likely diagnosis and why.

4. What diagnostic test or tests would you order and why?

He has had a postoperative echocardiogram that shows he has an ejection fraction (EF) of 30% with anterior wall hypokinesis. Chest x-ray shows a mild to moderate layering left chest effusion. There appears to also be a fracture of the upper sternal wire. His troponins are still elevated but decreasing.

5. Outline the treatment plan. Please tell me the initial treatment and next steps if that fails.

When his family arrives, more history becomes available. You discover he has a significant history of alcohol use, which was not recorded in the original history. He also is estranged from his family and lives in a single room in an apartment with two flights of stairs to enter, working as a bouncer at a local bar.

6. What are some of the potential obstacles to immediate rehabilitation and to eventual discharge? How will these affect the planned rehabilitation program?

As you are working to plan for discharge, the family states categorically that they will not take the patient into their home and that they are "not responsible for him." The only person who visits regularly and seems to be involved is a good friend, who works at the bar but appears to also be inebriated on several occasions when she visits the hospital.

7. Tell me what potential issues may be present in his discharge. How would you try to assure a stable discharge plan?

Answers

1. You will want to ask for his smoking and other risk factor history for the eventual lifestyle modification plan that may be required. In his hospitalization, you need to know the exact nature of the cardiac disease, any cardiac catheterization data, and the operative course. Specifically, you want to know the length of bypass time and the total time on bypass. If the cross camp time is significantly shorter than the total bypass time, that may indicate difficulty of coming off of bypass and indicate possible myocardial injury or a decreased EF. It is also essential to know if there was an actual infarct as well as if there are other known comorbidities. Often this is not able to be fully assessed and the social history also cannot be fully assessed in the initial acute admission due to the emergent nature of the hospitalization and treatment, so social history and prior functional status may only be available later during the hospitalization. It is essential to know the nature of the myocardial injury and the status of the heart to plan for inclusion of heart failure rehabilitation as well as postischemic injury rehabilitation, and to also assess what form the rehabilitation program will have. Assessing neurological status is also essential as up to 5% of bypass surgery patients can have strokes or other neurological injuries.

2. Physical exam can be done in the ICU and should be a complete exam with particular focus on some special elements. In patients with a median sternotomy, assessment of sternal stability is essential and can be done with palpation of the sternum under a palm feeling for a click (abnormal finding, there should be no click at all) or holding a flat palm on a sternum while the patient coughs as this can also elicit the click. Extremities need evaluation for deep vein thrombosis (DVT) and assessment of the vein donor sites, as well as a complete neurological exam to rule out peripheral nerve palsy injuries (brachial plexopathy and radial nerve and axillary nerve injuries are most common) as well as central nervous system injuries (mostly stroke, but spinal cord injury can rarely occur). Physical exam also will include the postoperative sternal wires and the chest tube if present. This will give an overall assessment of the status of the surgical recovery as well.

3. Several potential issues should present themselves: first is a possible sternal instability, which may indicate a broken sternal wire; the possible presence of a pleural effusion even with the chest tube in place; and a new anterior wall infarct, which may indicate the potential for a degree of heart failure.

4. A chest x-ray with lateral decubitus views will assess the sternal wires as well as the effusion. An echocardiogram can help assess ventricular function. Even if there is a reduction early, this may be temporary as there can be stunned myocardium that will now recover after reperfusion. Since there are no clear neurological findings, neurological imaging is not indicated.

5. Treatment should induce management of the effusion in conjunction with the surgical team and medical team. Thoracentesis or pericardiocentesis may

be needed if the effusion increases in the future (one in 2,000 cases). The goal for discharge is independent ambulation and ability to do about three to four metabolic equivalents (METs) of exercise. He needs to be independent with sit-to-stand and bed mobility without breaking sternal precautions. This is often more challenging than gait. Sternal precautions will need to be very strictly enforced in this individual. He may require repeat surgery to repair the sternal nonunion if this persists or is very bothersome. The low EF indicates a potential of significant myocardial injury and modification of the exercise protocol for heart failure can be done with modified exercise, long warm-up and cool down, and observation for overfatigue. The goal is to aim for a mobilization program at home with walking at a level of three to four METs. He should be referred for an outpatient cardiac rehabilitation program, which will need to start several weeks post-discharge. He will not be able to do full upper activities and will have sternal precautions for at least 6 weeks post-surgery, potentially longer with the early failure of a wire. Finally, he will need to start secondary prevention, which can start immediately with education. Using eighth-grade level language, go through the basics. Smoking cessation (if applicable) is a must. Weight loss is also essential. This is done through portion control and a diet low in sugar, starches, and saturated fat (the latter may need more explanation). Exercise will be taught in the cardiac rehabilitation program. Educate regarding high blood pressure, managing salt intake, and taking all medications including for blood pressure, lipid lowering, antiplatelet activity, and heart rate control.

6. The additional component here is the social isolation from family and likely very poor lifestyle with his history of alcohol use. Getting to and from the rehabilitation as an outpatient may be hard, lifestyle modification can be challenging, and his occupation will not be able to be resumed for months as he cannot use his arms for any activities above 5 to 10 pounds. This will also require an alcohol cessation program; the delirium in the ICU may have been alcohol withdrawal. If he is a smoker, this will make smoking cessation even harder to achieve.

7. Social work will clearly need to help assess the stability of his living situation. His friend may be a good support, but this needs to be clarified and the patient will need to allow the friend to be brought into the management of his condition. The potential of alcohol use and poor lifestyle choices may make lifestyle changes hard to achieve. Other options, including looking at alternative career choices and help with a better living situation, can be explored as well as assuring a better environment to stop drinking and smoking, and lead a healthier lifestyle.

BIBLIOGRAPHY

Bartels MN, Prince D. Cardiac rehabilitation. In: Mitra R, ed., *Principles of Rehabilitation Medicine*. McGraw Hill Education; 2019:chap 49:868–882.

Prince DZ, Bartels MN. Exercise recommendations for older adults for prevention of disability. In: Cifu D, ed. *Textbook of Geriatric Rehabilitation*. Elsevier; 2018:chap 14. https://doi.org/10.1016/B978-0-323-54454-2.00014-5

Thomas RJ, Balady G, Banka G, et al. 2018 ACC/AHA clinical performance and quality measures for cardiac rehabilitation: a report of the American College of Cardiology/American Heart Association Task Force on Performance Measures. *J Am Coll Cardiol*. 2018;71(16):1814–1837. https://doi.org/10.1016/j.jacc.2018.01.004

Thomas RJ, King M, Lui K, et al. (Writing Committee to Develop Clinical Performance Measures for Cardiac Rehabilitation). AACVPR/ACCF/AHA 2010 update: performance measures on cardiac rehabilitation for referral to cardiac rehabilitation/secondary prevention services endorsed by the American College of Chest Physicians, the American College of Sports Medicine, the American Physical Therapy Association, the Canadian Association of Cardiac Rehabilitation, the Clinical Exercise Physiology Association, the European Association for Cardiovascular Prevention and Rehabilitation, the Inter-American Heart Foundation, the National Association of Clinical Nurse Specialists, the Preventive Cardiovascular Nurses Association, and the Society of Thoracic Surgeons. American Association of Cardiovascular and Pulmonary Rehabilitation; American College of Cardiology Foundation; American Heart Association Task Force on Performance Measures. *J Am Coll Cardiol.* 2010;56(14):1159–1167. https://doi.org/10.1016/j.jacc.2010.06.006

A 63-year-old woman with no heart attack, but just treated with an outpatient angioplasty for single-vessel coronary disease, is referred for outpatient cardiac rehabilitation. She is presenting for initial evaluation 3 days after the angioplasty.

Questions

1. What more do you want to know about the patient's history, comorbidities, and social situation? Please tell me why you are asking for these specifics.

2. How would you go about performing a physical exam on this patient? Why are these maneuvers/exam components important?

You learn of a significant family history with both parents affected and also an older brother. She has multiple lifestyle issues including obesity, smoking, sedentary lifestyle, and early menopause. She has cholesteatoma and has severe arthritis in her knees. You find that she also has mild peripheral vascular disease (PVD) with an ankle-brachial index (ABI) of 0.90. Her sensation is intact and her neurologic exam is normal. Cardiac exam is also normal.

3. What is the differential diagnosis for this patient? Tell me the most likely diagnosis and why.

4. What diagnostic test or tests would you order and why?

A review of her lab data shows a normal cardiogram and an echocardiogram with EF of 55%, normal valve function. Catheterization data shows single vessel occlusion of the circumflex with patent graft after bare-metal stent. She has total cholesterol of 300 with low-density lipoprotein (LDL) 180. Body mass index (BMI) is 32.4, with normal blood chemistries and normal complete blood count (CBC).

5. Outline the treatment plan. Please tell me the initial treatment and next steps if that fails.

At the end of your visit, after you explain the classical 3-month cardiac rehabilitation program, she reveals that she has lost her job and her insurance will end in 1 month. She has no other insurance coverage and does not have the resources to pay for cardiac rehabilitation out of pocket.

6. How care might be facilitated?

She will start cardiac rehabilitation and secondary prevention. You will enroll her in smoking cessation and a nutritionally-guided weight loss program. However, the smoking and weight loss programs will not have openings for more than 1 month. How do you proceed with weight loss and smoking cessation?

7. Tell me in lay terms how you would provide assistance in managing her smoking and weight loss issues.

Answers

1. A complete review of systems focusing on the cardiovascular system with emphasis on claudication, stroke, and other vascular issues is important as atherosclerosis is often a systemic disease. Lifestyle history including smoking and diet history as well as activity history are important. There should also be a screen for depression or anxiety, as these are common in individuals with heart disease. The major challenge is that the patients will need to be made to start exercisong and often this has not been a lifestyle choice in the past, so assessing resistance to change can be partially assessed in the history.

2. Physical exam should look for stigmata of PVD and also assess for overall fitness and ability to perform exercise in elderly patients or patients with a history of significant debilitating disease, a frailty assessment may also be indicated. Look for decreased peripheral pulses, stigmata of elevated cholesterol such as xanthelasma or arcus senilis, and other signs of vascular disease as appropriate. Of course, a complete cardiovascular exam is also indicted; for example, listening for carotid bruits or fundoscopic exam in diabetics.

3. Diagnoses in addition to the coronary artery disease includes PVD. There may also be renal insufficiency or other conditions. She is a smoker and this is a risk factor that will need to be addressed, along with being obese.

4. If not available, a baseline EKG will be indicated as well as noninvasive flow studies to assess her peripheral circulation. An echocardiogram, if not already done, may be helpful as well. A baseline exercise test with a 6-minute walk or other field test can help design an exercise program. Defining her hypercholesterolemia and then working to improve her blood lipids in coordination with her primary care or cardiology team will also be useful.

5. She will start cardiac rehabilitation and secondary prevention. You will enroll her in smoking cessation and a nutritionally-guided weight loss program. If she is diabetic, podiatric care for her feet is also indicated. Smoking cessation and weight control will be the hardest secondary prevention issues and will need to be addressed together, as many individuals who stop smoking gain weight.

6. This is a challenge in cardiac rehabilitation. Although it is covered by all insurance plans, access can be a challenge and for may insurance plans, the copayments for cardiac rehabilitation sessions can be as high as $40 per session, leading to expenditures of $120 a week (or $1,440 for a complete program) on top of travel costs in individuals who have often just lost employment and are on a fixed income. Social work services are of great importance in helping here. For this patient, as she is 63 years old, she may be eligible for Medicare and/or Medicaid if she retires now.

7. Starting the smoking cessation as soon as possible is essential, and assistance with abstinence can help with pharmacological interventions. This can be medications in combination with nicotine replacement as well as counseling. Counseling for nutrition should include portion control as well as avoidance of animal fats and processed carbohydrates. Since weight gain may occur with smoking cessation, simultaneous weight counseling would be the best course. Motivational interviewing may also have a role, as it has been shown to be more effective than lecturing. Assess her readiness to change. Ask her what the barriers are to smoking cessation and weight loss. Address these together by problem-solving.

BIBLIOGRAPHY

Balady GJ, Williams MA, Ades PA, et al. Core components of cardiac rehabilitation/secondary prevention programs: 2007 update: a scientific statement from the American Heart Association Exercise, Cardiac Rehabilitation, and Prevention Committee, the Council on Clinical Cardiology; the Councils on Cardiovascular Nursing, Epidemiology and Prevention, and Nutrition, Physical Activity, and Metabolism; and the American Association of Cardiovascular and Pulmonary Rehabilitation. *Circulation.* May 22, 2007;115(20):2675–2682. https://doi.org/10.1161/CIRCULATIONAHA.106.180945

Bartels MN. Cardiopulmonary rehabilitation. In: Batmangelich S, ed. *Physical Medicine and Rehabilitation Patient-Centered Care.* Demos Publishing; 2014:112–129. https://doi.org/10.1891/9781617051333.0011

Bartels MN, Prince D. Cardiac rehabilitation. In: Mitra R, ed., *Principles of Rehabilitation Medicine.* McGraw Hill Education; 2019:chap 49:868–882

Piepoli MF, Corra U, Adamopoulos S, et al. Secondary prevention in the clinical management of patients with cardiovascular diseases. Core components, standards and outcome measures for referral and delivery: a policy statement from the cardiac rehabilitation section of the European Association for Cardiovascular Prevention & Rehabilitation. Endorsed by the Committee for Practice Guidelines of the European Society of Cardiology. *Eur J Prev Cardiol.* June 2014;21(6):664–681. https://doi.org/10.1177/2047487312449597

Prince DZ, Bartels MN. Exercise recommendations for older adults for prevention of disability. In: Cifu D, ed. *Textbook of Geriatric Rehabilitation.* Elsevier; 2018:chap 14. https://doi.org/10.1016/B978-0-323-54454-2.00014-5

CASE 3

A 67-year-old man with diabetes and a vague history of cardiac disease is referred to the physical medicine and rehabilitation (PM&R) clinic by his general internist because of claudication and gait difficulty. He was diagnosed with angina 4 years ago and treated medically with medications (beta-blockade, aspirin, and nitrates). He was also started on lipid-lowering medications and told to improve his diabetic control, but he has not been as compliant with his regimen as could be desired. In addition, he has continued to smoke. He presents for evaluation.

Questions

1. What more do you want to know about the patient's history, comorbidities, and social situation? Please tell me why you are asking for these specifics.

2. How would you go about performing a physical exam on this patient? Why are these maneuvers/exam components important?

His vascular symptoms include pain with walking for more than one block, and he has had no resting pain. These symptoms have been gradually worsening over the last 5 years. He does state that his feet are numb and he has more difficulty with walking uphill and walking quickly. He has not had any falls and there is no history of skin ulcers. He does report dry skin and has had some edema. Of note, he has no history of chest pain or shortness of breath and has no clear heart disease beyond what he reports as some "heart troubles" a few years ago. His blood pressure is normal. He has no skin ulcerations, but has absent pulses and has trophic skin changes. He has decreased sensation and also has foot fungus at the toenails with poor toenail hygiene. There is some mild peripheral hand muscle wasting with atrophic intrinsic hand muscles. His ABI is 0.55.

3. What is the differential diagnosis for this patient? Tell me the most likely diagnosis and why.

4. What diagnostic test or tests would you order and why?

His blood tests reveal elevated cholesterol with an elevated LDL, elevated hemoglobin A1c (HgA1c), and normal erythrocyte sedimentation rate (ESR) and CBC. EKG shows evidence of an old inferior wall myocardial infarction (MI) and normal sinus rhythm.

5. Outline the treatment plan. Please tell me initial treatment and next steps if that fails.

Unfortunately, the patient lives in a rural community and is 65 miles away from the closest rehabilitation program, which has a 5-month waiting list for their oversubscribed vascular rehabilitation program. The patient also has transportation challenges to attending a 3-day-a-week program.

6. How might care be facilitated? Are there treatment alternatives?

The final challenge is that the patient is a practicing Amish farmer and does not have access to the Internet or any modern technologies that would allow for a telemedicine or other remote option for care.

7. How would you resolve this conflict? What are the options for providing care to this patient in a remote area with no access to remote communication technology?

Answers

1. Ask about the course/timing of symptoms—leg/resting pain, numbness, functional limitations, chest pain, and shortness of breath—and perform a complete review of systems. Also consider a neurologic exam, as stroke is a comorbid condition.

2. On the physical exam, check for: muscle wasting, loss of muscle strength, alteration of sensation, abnormal blood pressure, cardiac abnormalities, decreased peripheral pulses, skin breakdown, or trophic skin changes. Consider ABI, a test to be done in the office. You could also do a step test or 6-minute walk test as field screening tests. Close assessment of the condition of toenails and footwear is indicated to prevent the formation of skin ulceration.

3. The differential is whether this is large-vessel or small-vessel PVD or a combination of the two. Most likely, this is PVD that has elements of small vessel diabetic vasculopathy as well as large vessel occlusive disease. The differential diagnosis list also includes peripheral neuropathy (diabetic), vascular insufficiency, comorbid cardiac ischemic disease, and comorbid chronic obstructive pulmonary disease (COPD).

4. Consider ABI, a test to be done in the office. You could also do a step test or 6-minute walk test as field screening tests. Noninvasive flow studies will also help to clearly define the extent of PVD in the individual. Close assessment of the condition of toenails and footwear is indicated to prevent the formation of skin ulceration. Differential: PVD, peripheral neuropathy (diabetic), vascular insufficiency, comorbid cardiac ischemic disease, comorbid COPD. Lab work should include lipid profile, HbA1C, CBC, ESR, and EKG.

5. He has significant PVD and also has evidence of old MI. This will complicate his treatment regimen as he will be at risk of ischemia with mobilization. Exercise therapy is recommended, as well as smoking cessation and secondary prevention with education, lifestyle modification, and diabetic teaching. Fortunately, the secondary preventive measures for cardiac disease and PVD overlap and the exercise program for both will help both the vascular disease as well as any occult ischemic heart disease. Exercise will include aerobic training focused on ambulation. Heart rate precautions will be 20 beats per minute (BPM) above resting heart rate (on beta-blocker) if no exercise test can be arranged. Strengthening exercises as well as postural and balance training will be appropriate. He will benefit from cardiac evaluation only if not recently done. Monitoring will be optional, but nice if available. He is at risk for foot ulcers and amputation. He should be trained to monitor his feet and may need a podiatrist. He should have regular eye exams for retinopathy. He is at risk for coronary disease and should be instructed about signs and symptoms of angina.

6. Remote and telemedicine solutions for vascular rehabilitation are not yet robust and readily available, but remote monitoring of an exercise program could be done using wearable heart rate monitors and step/distance counters. A moderate exercise program with walking can be done and there are many secondary educational resources available regarding lifestyle modifications that can be accessed via the Internet. This is unfortunately a common issue and has no easy solutions. Assessing if the patient is a veteran can add access to Veterans Affairs (VA) resources, but these are often also very limited in availability.

7. Using written materials is one aspect that can be done, and counseling remotely if possible. However, the scenario presented is an individual who would not have any electronic communication, including telephone, and would do not be likely to use modern remote monitoring devices. Having a general conditioning exercise program with written instructions may be the only option. Working up to a **1- to 2-mile-a-day** walking program and lifestyle counseling can provide the best solution.

BIBLIOGRAPHY

Hamburg NM, Balady GJ. Exercise rehabilitation in peripheral artery disease: functional impact and mechanisms of benefits. *Circulation.* 2011;123:87–97. https://doi.org/10.1161/CIRCULATIONAHA.109.881888

Peripheral arterial disease exercise training toolkit. AACVPR resources. https://www.aacvpr.org/Portals/0/Resources/PAD%20Toolkit/pad-exercise-training-toolkit_website.pdf

Writing Committee to Develop Guidelines for the Management of Patients With Peripheral Arterial Disease. ACC/AHA guidelines for the management of patients with peripheral arterial disease (lower extremity, renal, mesenteric, and abdominal aortic): executive summary: a collaborative report from the American Association for Vascular Surgery/Society for Vascular Surgery, Society for Cardiovascular Angiography and Interventions, Society for Vascular Medicine and Biology, Society of Interventional Radiology, and the ACC/AHA Task Force on Practice Guidelines. *J Am Coll Cardiol.* 2006;1:1–17.

A 68-year-old man with a 40 packs/year history of smoking with severe respira-tory failure was admitted to the ICU and intubated. You are called to assess him in the ICU for rehabilitation. He is currently awake on the ventilator, but unable to be weaned.

Questions

1. What more do you want to know about the patient's history, comor-bidities, and social situation? Please tell me why you are asking for these specifics.

2. How would you go about performing a physical exam on this patient? Why are these maneuvers/exam components important?

He has a history of smoking and was otherwise well until his admission. He has no clear history of cardiac disease and has had no cardiac issues since admission. He has no history of neurological or vascular disease. He is very thin but has good strength on individual muscle testing. Lung exam shows much-re-duced breath sounds. He has hyperreflexia and tachycardia with normal blood pressure. There are no focal motor or neurological findings.

3. What is the differential diagnosis for this patient? Tell me the most likely diagnosis and why.

4. What diagnostic test or tests would you order and why?

Chest x-ray has right lower lobe pneumonia but shows very reduced lung mark-ings. Once he is extubated, you find out he has severe obstructive pulmonary disease with a high residual volume and elevated total lung capacity on pulmo-nary function tests. EKG has right ventricular and atrial enlargement with a mild right axis deviation, and there is mild evidence of right ventricular enlargement on echocardiogram.

5. Outline the treatment plan. Please tell me the initial treatment and next steps if that fails.

When you are able to review his old medical records, you find he was treated for knee arthritis in the rehabilitation clinic a year and a half ago. The physical therapy program was ended early as he was unable to complete the recom-mended exercise programs due to fatigue and shortness of breath. The team never pursued the cause of that dyspnea.

6. Describe a quality improvement project to help address this potential issue.

Wanting to accelerate the course of this patient's recovery, you prescribe physical therapy and early mobilization for the patient even though he was still on the ventilator. The ICU staff and the intensive care director push back and refuse to allow the therapy to start until the patient is discharged from the ICU, stating it is too dangerous and would cause too much of a care burden.

7. Tell me in lay terms how you would resolve this conflict?

Answers

1. A complete history of respiratory exposures including occupational and smoking history as well as illicit drug use (marijuana, smoked cocaine, or heroin) should be obtained. Current functional status before admission should be acquired, along with cardiac and cancer risk history. The likelihood of cancer or other comorbidity is raised by his cachectic body habits and he might have significant comorbidities from other conditions

2. Exam can be done on the patient while in the ICU. This needs to also include lowering sedation if possible so a good neurological examination can be done. As with all patients in the ICU, the history and physical may be done over days as the patient is eventually improved and more exams can be done. Particular attention has to be paid to looking for skin breakdown and other complications of being in the ICU.

3. Prevention of the complications of immobility needs to be addressed (DVT, skin, urinary tract infection, pulmonary) as well as starting early mobilization in the ICU which will continue on the regular floor. The differential diagnosis will include emphysema and COPD, acute community-acquired pneumonia, postobstructive pneumonia with cancer, and pulmonary vascular disease. Most likely diagnosis is COPD with community-acquired pneumonia; many COPD patients are undiagnosed until they present with pulmonary failure. The hyperreflexia and tachycardia are likely due to beta-agonists and a hyper-adrenergic state and may not need to indicate cardiac or neurologic disease.

4. Chest x-ray and chest CT will help in the acute setting. Once off of the ventilator, pulmonary function tests and an echocardiogram will be helpful to diagnose the nature of the pulmonary disease and to rule out pulmonary hypertension and right ventricular failure. Eventually, an exercise test will help to assess functioning capacity. Arterial blood gas (ABG) can also be useful if there is drowsiness or other sedation (he may be hypercarbic on the supplemental oxygen or hypoxemic).

5. Patient needs to start early mobilization to prevent reconditioning and loss of strength, help with extubation, and decrease the length of his ICU stay. He has no history of pulmonary rehabilitation and needs to start with goals of education and secondary prevention along with medication education, as well as disease management and oxygen use education. Supplemental oxygen with exercise will likely be needed. Low flow oxygen can improve quality of life, prevent hospitalizations, and decrease mortality in patients with COPD. He will need a full assessment of his pulmonary and physical status as well once he is out of the ICU and off the ventilator. Once discharged from the hospital, he will need an outpatient pulmonary rehabilitation program. Goals are secondary prevention, smoking cessation, family and patient education, home exercise program, and a pulmonary rehabilitation program with strengthening and conditioning. Monitoring will be for vital signs and O_2

saturation. Precautions include heart rate and blood pressure (especially dia-stolic ceilings), as well as maintaining oxygen saturation above 90%. Finally, medication education and training in inhalers and oxygen management need to be done

6. Unfortunately, missing associated diagnoses are not all that uncommon. When we are treating patients, we need to be careful to not put on blinders and miss potentially serious other conditions. A simple spirometry test could have been performed to screen these patients for pulmonary disease earlier in their course. Then referral could have been made for pulmonary care or a notation to the primary care physician may have helped to identify their lung condition earlier and that may have allowed primary prevention to be done. A quality program for this could be to be sure that a review of systems is done and any positive findings that are not being treated or diagnosed could be noted. Any failures to complete a therapy program should be assessed to be sure no loose ends are left in patient care.

7. The best solution to the hesitance for early mobilization is to have open com-munication and be knowledgeable about the process. Start the communica-tion with the care team before a patient is admitted to the ICU so that the care providers are all in agreement. Early mobilization is safe and effective and should be done for all patients for whom it can be safely done. Familiarize yourself with the scientific literature that supports early mobilization in the ICU to reduce mortality, morbidity, and costs. Engage the ICU physicians in this. Work with hospital administration to assign physical therapists to the ICU, and educate the therapists regarding the feasibility of getting patients to exercise and mobilize while still ventilated. Establish guidelines for safe mobilization in terms of cardiopulmonary stability.

BIBLIOGRAPHY

Bartels MN, Bach J. Rehabilitation of the patient with respiratory dysfunction. In: Frontera W, Silver J, Rizzo T, ed. *Essentials of Rehabilitation*. 6th ed. Wolters Kluwer Health; 2019:chap 150:860–867.

Bartels MN, Prince DZ. Acute medical conditions. In: Cifu DX, ed. *Braddom's Physical Medicine and Rehabilitation*. 5th ed. Elsevier; 2015:571–595.

Cameron S, Ball I, Cepinskas G, et al. Early mobilization in the critical care unit: a review of adult and pediatric literature [Review]. *J Crit Care*. August 2015;30(4):664–672. https://doi.org/10.1016/j.jcrc.2015.03.032

Kruis AL, Smidt N, Assendelft WJ, et al. Integrated disease management interventions for patients with chronic obstruc-tive pulmonary disease [Review]. *Cochrane Database Syst Rev*. 2013;10:CD009437. https://doi.org/10.1002/14651858. CD009437.pub2

CASE 5

A 58-year-old nurse is admitted to the hospital with a COVID-19 infection acquired from either the community or at work. She is in respiratory distress and intubated. After a 4-week ICU course, she is finally extubated and discharged from the ICU to the step-down unit. You are asked to do a rehabilitation evaluation.

Questions

1. What more do you want to know about the patient's history, comorbidities, and social situation? Please tell me why you are asking for these specifics.

2. How would you go about performing a physical exam on this patient? Why are these maneuvers/exam components important?

She had no pulmonary issues in the past and was working full time as part of the nursing staff. She had a history of mild hypertension, no cardiac disease, no PVD, and no neurological or cardiac disease. Her hospitalization was notable for respiratory failure with interstitial lung disease, cardiomyopathy with a decreased EF, and slow recovery from sedation used while intubated. She is a chronically ill-looking woman, frail, and tachypneic on high flow (6 L) nasal cannula oxygen. She has marked muscle wasting, and there are several skin breakdowns. She has left-hand weakness on exam and no other clear neurological findings. Her mental status is clear, but she is mildly distractible and has poor concentration. Pulmonary exam is notable for bilateral crackles at the bases.

3. What is the differential diagnosis for this patient? Tell me the most likely diagnosis and why.

4. What additional diagnostic test or tests would you order and why?

Pulmonary function tests show marked restrictive lung disease with a very low diffusion for carbon monoxide (DLCO). She has marked hypoxemia with pO_2 of only 86 mmHg on 6 L of oxygen via nasal cannula. Chest CT with marked increase of interstitial markings in all lung fields. Echocardiogram has an EF of 45%. Electromyography is consistent with critical illness myopathy and neuropathy with a radial nerve palsy, and head CT is normal.

5. Outline the treatment plan. Please tell me the initial treatment and next steps.

In the surge of COVID-19 patients, the inpatient rehabilitation unit has been transformed into a unit for treating acutely ill COVID-19 patients. With her youth and the hope that she can be restored to a sufficiently recovered state that she might get a lung transplant, you are caught in a situation where there may not be any available acute rehabilitation resources to admit the patient, and the acute hospital needs to have her move to the next level of post-acute care.

6. How might care might be facilitated? How can you address the ethical dilemma?

The patient is evaluated for possible lung transplantation by the lung transplant team. As a part of the evaluation, it appears that she has an undiagnosed breast mass and is found to have stage 1 breast cancer. She will need to be disease-free for 2 years before lung transplant might be possible, but has such severe lung disease that mortality is expected to be 50% within a year.

7. Please describe, in lay terms, the rehabilitation approach to the patient and her family that will achieve the best quality of life while understanding that it may be hard to achieve the needed 2-year cancer-free survival with her current severe pulmonary disease?

Answers

1. The key elements of the history to find out are the hospital course, the prior functional status, and the history of pulmonary and extrapulmonary disease. Although COVID-19 is a brand new condition and is not fully characterized, it appears to be a multisystemic disease. There are clear central nervous system issues including stroke delirium and encephalopathy, a diffuse vasculopathy with multiple complications in eluding excess skin breakdown, and cardiomyopathy, just to name a few. Social support for a prolonged recovery is important as well.

2. The exam needs to include a full medical and neurological exam. Special attention should be paid to a complete skin exam, neurological exam to rule out neuropathy and central nervous system injury, and cardiopulmonary exam. A 6-minute walk test or other frailty examinations such as a timed up and go test can be done to assess for frailty as many patients, even younger ones, have significant systemic weakness and muscle loss in recovery from COVID-19.

3. Differential includes critical illness myopathy, critical illness neuropathy, stroke, brachial plexopathy or peripheral neuropathy, delirium, and encephalopathy.

4. There might be a role for electromyography and head CT scan, and for the cardiac and pulmonary disease, echocardiography and chest CT. Categorizing functional capacity may include a functional exercise test.

5. Treatment will include early mobilization with a focus on reducing post-intensive care syndrome (PICS). Gentle strengthening as well as full nutritional and psychological support need to be done. Skin care for breakdown as well as prevention of other breakdown. For the neuropathy, appropriate nutrition will need to be assured and protection from complications with appropriate treatment as needed for dysesthesias. The pulmonary disease will require a comprehensive pulmonary rehabilitation program. High flow supplemental oxygen will be needed for mobilization because of her severe interstitial lung disease. The goal is to use as much oxygen as needed to maintain the oxygen saturation above 90% with therapy. The role of anticoagulation for prevention of DVT will also be important, as COVID-19 is associated with excess thrombotic events and pulmonary embolisms. Assessment for lung transplantation may be indicated as it appears severe lung injury from COVID-19 may not recover and the patient's only option may be transplantation.

6. There is no single answer or a correct answer in this situation. When presented with a patient with so many rehabilitation needs, it is clear that acute inpatient rehabilitation would be best. However, in the surge or in many other situations, the resources may not be available. And in a crisis, there may need to be suboptimal discharge plans as the acute care beds are needed for more unstable patients. Creating a comprehensive program for rehabilitation

in a skilled nursing facility or fighting to keep the patient in the acute care setting while providing more therapy may be options. Working with hospital administration to find the best solutions while also managing the care team, patient, and family expectations is essential. This will require diplomacy and a firm defense of the best interests of your patient.

7. Unfortunately, situations like this are not uncommon in transplantation rehabilitation. The added twist of COVID-19 does not change the underlying tension between promoting patients for transplantation while avoiding known issues for excess mortality. Creating realistic expectations as well as planning a rehabilitation program on maintaining quality of life while maintaining function is essential for a successful bridging to transplantation. It is important to remember that while pulmonary rehabilitation may decrease exacerbations and admissions, it may not clearly be associated with improved survival. However, the maintenance of strength and conditioning through rehabilitation can allow a patient to remain an active candidate for transplantation over a longer period, since very weak or sarcopenic patients cannot be transplanted. This will require close work with the patient, the family, and the transplant team.

BIBLIOGRAPHY

Ambrose AF, Bartels MN, Verghese TC, et al. Patient and caregiver guide to managing COVID-19 patients at home. *J Int Soc Phys Rehabil Med.* 2020;3:53–68. https://doi.org/10.4103/jisprm.jisprm_4_20 (epub ahead of print: April 15, 2020).

Bartels MN, Bach J. Rehabilitation of the patient with respiratory dysfunction. In: Frontera W, Silver J, Rizzo T, ed. *Essentials of Rehabilitation.* 6th ed. Wolters Kluwer Health.Wolters Kluwer Health; 2019:chap 150:860–867.

Gitkind AI, Levin S, Dohle C, et al. Redefining pathways into acute rehabilitation during the COVID-19 crisis. *PM R.* August 2020;12(8):837–841. April 29. https://doi.org/10.1002/pmrj.12392. Online ahead of print.

Lopez M, Bell K, Annaswamy T, et al. COVID-19 guide for the rehabilitation clinician: a review of non-pulmonary manifestations and complications. *Am J Phys Med Rehabil.* 2020;99(8):669–673, 8. https://doi.org/10.1097/PHM.0000000000001479

Yonter SJ, Alter K, Bartels MN, et al. What now for rehabilitation specialists? Coronavirus disease 2019 (COVID-19) questions and answers. *Arch Phys Med Rehabil.* 2020;101:2233-2242. https://doi.org/10.1016/j.apmr.2020.09.368

5 Complex Medical Rehabilitation

R. Samuel Mayer

A 33-year-old transgender person identifying as female with HIV is referred to the physical medicine and rehabilitation (PM&R) clinic by her infectious disease specialist because of weakness and fatigue. She was diagnosed 4 years ago and was started on highly active antiretroviral therapy (HAART) therapy. She has not been compliant with this regimen. Her CD4 count last month was 250/mm (normal >500/mm), and her viral load was 10,000 copies (normal undetectable).

Questions

1. What more do you want to know about the patient's history, comorbidities, and social situation? Please tell me why you are asking for these specifics.

2. How would you go about performing a physical exam on this patient? Why are these maneuvers/exam components important?

You learn her weakness is generalized, began about 1 month ago, and has been progressive. She reports muscle aches and fatigue. She has had HIV for 15 years. She started hormonal therapy 2 years ago and has not had gender reassignment surgery yet. She has difficulty arising from a chair and climbing stairs. Her knees buckle with prolonged standing or walking more than a block. She has lost about 5 kg (10 lb.) this month. She has no fevers, numbness, headaches, diplopia, dysphagia, or bowel or bladder incontinence. She is on Biktarvy for her HIV, and spironolactone for testosterone suppression, as well as transdermal estrogen. Vials are normal and she is not orthostatic. Body mass index (BMI) is 18. She has no cranial nerve deficits. She has muscle wasting and 4/5 strength in her proximal muscles; distally she is 5/5. Reflexes are normal. Sensation is intact. Range of motion is full in all four limbs and the spine. There is no vertebral tenderness.

3. What is the differential diagnosis for this patient? Tell me the most likely diagnosis and why.

4. What diagnostic test or tests would you order and why?

Creatine kinase (CK) and C-reactive protein (CRP) are normal. Electromyography (EMG)/nerve conduction study (NCS) shows normal NCS and low-amplitude polyphasic motor unit potentials (MUPs) without spontaneous activity.

5. Outline the treatment plan. Please tell me the initial treatment and next steps if that fails.

The patient reports that she has been very depressed.

6. How would you address this?

At the conclusion of your visit, she reports that she is unemployed and sometimes resorts to prostitution.

7. How would you discuss this issue with her?

Answers

1. How is this impacting her function? Activities of daily living (ADLs) and work? How long has she felt weak? Does she have any change in sensation? What medications does she take? Does she have any fevers, weight loss, headaches, visual changes, difficulty swallowing, or bowel or bladder dysfunction?

2. Check vitals, including orthostatics. Observe for muscle wasting. Check cranial nerves, sensation, strength, and coordination.

3. Differential diagnosis includes HIV sarcopenia, neuropathy, brain abscess (particularly toxoplasmosis), epidural abscess, and adrenal insufficiency. Biktarvy and spironolactone can cause muscle cramps, but not usually weakness. Sarcopenia is the most likely diagnosis given the lack of upper motor neuron signs, sensory loss, and lack of orthostasis.

4. CK and EMG may help establish myopathy. CRP can help rule out infectious or inflammatory etiologies. MRI of the brain and spinal cord could be considered if more focal signs were present.

5. An exercise program including strength training is likely the most effective treatment. Compliance with antiviral medications also will help. While testosterone has been used in treating HIV sarcopenia, it would be contraindicated in this transgender woman.

6. Depression and suicidal ideation are extremely common in transgender individuals. Ask her if she has any thoughts of hurting herself. Ask about vegetative symptoms. Referral to psychology or psychiatry may be indicated. There are also excellent support groups for transgender individuals.

7. First, the physician should ask how this person likes to be addressed, especially regarding pronouns. Lay terms (eighth-grade level) should be used to explain things. Ask the patient about employment history, academic background and skills to elucidate other vocational options. Recognize the major role that prejudice plays in transgender persons lives, including employment discrimination. Obviously, prostitution carries a heavy risk of HIV transmission, and a nonjudgmental discussion about how she might inform clients and about use of condoms should be had.

BIBLIOGRAPHY

Bonato M, Turrini F, Galli L, et al. The role of physical activity for the management of Sarcopenia in people living with HIV. *Int J Environ Res Public Health.* 2020;17(4):1283. Published 2020 Feb 17. https://doi.org/10.3390/ijerph17041283

Hembree WC, Cohen-Kettenis PT, Gooren L, et al. Endocrine treatment of gender-dysphoric/gender-incongruent persons: an endocrine society clinical practice guideline. *J Clin Endocrinol Metab.* 2017;102:3869. https://doi.org/10.1210/jc.2017-01658

Weyers S, Elaut E, De Sutter P, et al. Long-term assessment of the physical, mental, and sexual health among transsexual women. *J Sex Med.* 2009;6:752. https://doi.org/10.1111/j.1743-6109.2008.01082.x

CASE 2

You are consulted in the ICU on a 65-year-old man who is now intubated on mechanical ventilation due to COVID-19 severe acute respiratory syndrome (SARS). You are asked to identify future rehabilitation needs.

Questions

1. What more do you want to know about the patient's history, comorbidities, and social situation? Please tell me why you are asking for these specifics.

2. How would you go about performing a physical exam on this patient? Why are these maneuvers/exam components important?

He was diagnosed with COVID-19 3 weeks ago, and has been on the ventilator for 10 days; he is scheduled for tracheostomy and gastrostomy tube placement tomorrow. Per nursing, he "sun-downs" in the evenings and gets agitated, so they have to use mitts to keep him from pulling out his tubes. He has a past history of chronic obstructive pulmonary disease (COPD) from tobacco abuse, obesity, and type 2 diabetes mellitus (DM). He is retired and lives with his wife, who is also retired, and an adult son who is working from home. The home has two stories with bedrooms and baths upstairs.

On exam, his vitals are stable and he is on intermittent mandatory ventilation and has begun spontaneous breathing trials. He is alert and communicates by writing. He is oriented to person and place but not date. His Mini-Mental State Exam is 20/30. He has crackles at the lung bases; heart is regular rate and rhythm. He has a benign abdominal exam. He has 1+ edema but no calf tenderness. Cranial nerves are intact. He has poor proprioception. Strength is 4/5 in his hands and ankles and is 5/5 elsewhere. Babinski and Hoffman signs are negative, and reflexes are 1+ throughout.

3. What is the differential diagnosis for this patient's cognitive dysfunction and weakness? Tell me the most likely diagnosis and why.

4. What diagnostic test or tests would you order and why?

MRI and electrodiagnostic studies could not be done in the COVID ICU. His complete blood count (CBC), comprehensive metabolic panel (CMP), ammonia level, lactate, B12, thyroid-stimulating hormone (TSH), and rapid plasma reagin (RPR) are normal; blood sugars have ranged from 100 to 175. A videofluoroscopy swallow study shows aspiration of all food and fluid consistencies.

5. Outline the ICU rehab program.

Ten days later, the patient has weaned off the ventilator and is medically stable on a general medicine unit. Repeat COVID-19 test is negative. The medical team would like to move him to rehabilitation.

6. What criteria would you use to determine his appropriate level of rehab care? For the purpose of this question, assume the patient has Medicare and a Medi-gap insurance.

You inform the patient's wife that he is moving to the rehabilitation unit. However, the rehab unit has a no-visitor policy due to COVID-19 precautions (as did the acute care floor). She is quite angry about this and demands to be able to see her husband.

7. What would you say to the wife to allay her concerns?

Answers

1. When was he diagnosed and how long has he been in the ICU? What is his respiratory status? Has he had complications? What comorbidities does he have? What is his living situation?

2. Listen to lungs for crackles and the heart for arrhythmia. Check the calves for tenderness as COVID patients are at high risk for deep venous thrombosis (DVT). Do a thorough neuro exam.

3. His weakness is probably ICU neuropathy, but he could also have preexisting diabetic neuropathy. He may have steroid myopathy, as most COVID patients receive dexamethasone. He likely has ICU delirium. Lacunar strokes are common in COVID patients. One would also want to rule out other reversible causes of delirium and weakness, including sepsis, B12 deficiency, hypoglycemia, hypothyroidism, neurosyphilis, electrolyte abnormalities, and high ammonia levels. Review his medications for those with possible psychotropic side effects.

4. While MRI and electrodiagnostic tests would be helpful, this is not likely to be available in a COVID unit. Lab work could include CBC, CMP, lactate, ammonia, B12, TSH, and RPR.

5. For his delirium, frequent reorientation, restoration of sleep–wake cycles, elimination of any CNS active meds as possible, and minimization of unnecessary tubes and restraints would help. Speech pathology would treat his dysphagia, tracheostomy care, and cognitive issues. Occupational therapy (OT) can start with simple ADLs. Physical therapy (PT) can mobilize him, and even walk with him using a portable ventilator. He is likely to have tachycardia and tachypnea with exertion, and you should implement reasonable precautions for this (e.g., heart rate <75% maximal). All staff should utilize proper personal protective equipment.

6. To come to a comprehensive integrated rehabilitation program, he should be medically stable enough that he no longer requires diagnostic testing that would substantially interfere with his therapy schedule. While normally he would have to tolerate and benefit from greater than 3 hours of PT, OT, and speech-language pathology (SLP) daily, at the time of this writing, Medicare has waived that requirement due to COVID limitations.

7. Express empathy with the wife's situation and how stressful it must be not to be able to visit personally. Explain the rationale for the visitor restrictions to protect her and other patients. Offer video visits if feasible, as well as reassure her that the rehab team will update her daily.

BIBLIOGRAPHY

Simpson R, Robinson L. Rehabilitation after critical illness in people with COVID-19 infection. *Am J Phys Med Rehabil.* 2020;99(6):470–474. https://doi.org/10.1097/PHM.0000000000001443

Trogrli Z, van der Jagt M, Bakker J, et al. A systematic review of implementation strategies for assessment, prevention, and management of ICU delirium and their effect on clinical outcomes. *Crit Care.* 2015;19(1):157. https://doi.org/10.1186/s13054-015-0886-9

Vanhorebeek I, Latronico N, Van den Berghe G. ICU-acquired weakness. *Intensive Care Med.* 2020;46(4):637–653. https://doi.org/10.1007/s00134-020-05944-4

6 Durable Medical Equipment

Brad E. Dicianno

A 34-year-old woman with lumbar level myelomeningocele presents for an assistive technology evaluation in an outpatient clinic. She is complaining of recurrent skin breakdown and is worried it is related to her wheelchair.

Questions

1. What key elements about her history would you need to elicit? Explain why you need to obtain this information.

2. What aspects of the physical exam will you collect? Explain why you will collect each component of the exam.

She uses a power wheelchair that is 2 years old and has had minor repair issues. She has tilt, recline, elevating leg rests, and a foam cushion. She does not use the seat functions regularly. She is on a bladder catheterization program and rarely incontinent of urine. However, she is incontinent of bowel, which has especially been an issue at work. Nutrition is good with adequate protein. She says that her transfers and pressure relief maneuvers are becoming difficult to conduct independently because of shoulder pain. She thinks this is contributing to some shear when she is transferring.

She required minimum assistance to transfer out of the wheelchair onto a mat table. She has a 2-cm, Stage II pressure injury on her right ischial tuberosity, with moderate serosanguineous drainage and clean borders. Stool incontinence is present. She had no appreciable scoliosis on her exam. She has 2/5 strength in the bilateral hip flexors but otherwise 0/5 strength in lower limbs. She has absent sensation in the L2 dermatome and below bilaterally.

3. What is the differential diagnosis for the skin breakdown? How did you arrive at this differential diagnosis?

4. What type of testing would you want to order?

Pressure mapping shows a significantly elevated area of pressure under the right ischial tuberosity.

5. Besides appropriate wound care, what other interventions would you propose to help heal the pressure injury?

Because incontinence is an issue, you would ideally like for her to have two incontinence covers for her cushion so that she could use one while the other is being cleaned. However, her insurance will not pay for an additional cover and she does not have a caregiver to help her clean her cushion.

6. How might you address this dilemma?

Due to her history of hydrocephalus, which causes impairments in executive function, she has a difficult time remembering all of the information you provided to her and says that she will have a difficult time remembering to keep the right amount of air in her cushion.

7. What might you do to help facilitate your plan for this patient?

Answers

1. You should obtain information that will elucidate the etiology of the skin breakdown and whether it may be related to her equipment. Ask about the type of wheelchair she uses (manual, power assist, or power), and, if she uses a power wheelchair, whether she currently has and uses any power seat functions. Also ask whether she can transfer or conduct pressure relief maneuvers independently. It would also be useful to know what type of cushion she uses. Ask the age of the equipment and whether it is in disrepair. Obtain review of system data regarding incontinence/moisture, nutrition status, and any potential sources of pressure and shear.

2. On her exam, determine the size, stage, location, and condition of any skin breakdown. Evaluate her ability to transfer in and out of the equipment. Evaluate her seating position to determine if scoliosis or any other factors might be contributing to seating asymmetries. Evaluate her sensation and motor function in the lower limbs. This information will help determine what factors are contributing to skin breakdown and what interventions may help address it.

3. The history and physical exam point to an etiology that is possibly multifactorial, from a combination of pressure, shear, and incontinence.

4. Pressure mapping should be ordered. This will allow you to visualize the extent to which pressure may be contributing to the wound and is an educational tool for the patient.

5. A new cushion is likely indicated, and ideally the selection of a cushion may depend on which demo cushion showed the best pressure distribution on pressure mapping. Generally, air or gel cushions provide better pressure relief than foam cushions. Tilt, combined with recline, offer the best pressure relief for this type of wound. The physiatrist should work with the therapist to determine if changes can be made to her seating positioning to reduce asymmetry in seating that might be causing more pressure on the right side. She may also benefit from physical therapy to treat shoulder pain and evaluate transfers. She would also benefit from a better bowel program to improve incontinence.

6. You can work with the supplier to identify the cost of the additional cover. If she wants an additional cover but cannot pay for it out of pocket, you should discuss other funding options with her, such as a vocational rehabilitation program. She may need accommodations at work to handle her bowel issues. She may also benefit from an attendant care program for caregiver assistance.

7. First, "do no harm." The principle of nonmaleficence is appropriate to apply here. Although an air cushion might provide good pressure relief, it might be difficult to maintain, and therefore cause harm to the patient. Choose a

cushion that provides good pressure relief but is also easy for her to maintain. She will require education on risk for skin breakdown and the fact that the causes are multifactorial. She will require education on the proper use of power seat functions. Transfer training may be warranted. Education about pressure and shear on other surfaces such as commodes or shower chairs may also be warranted. Her independence in self-management could be facilitated with cognitive aids such as electronic reminders, printed educational material that include pictures or checklists, and follow-up appointments to implement a step-by-step approach to the plan. A multidisciplinary approach with other members of the treatment team could be used to reinforce the information you want to provide.

BIBLIOGRAPHY

Cooper RA. Wheelchair adjustment and maintenance. In: Cooper RA, ed. *Wheelchair Selection and Configuration.* Demos Medical Publishing; 1998:371–390.

Dicianno BE, Lieberman J, Schmeler MR, et al. Rehabilitation engineering and assistive technology society of North America's position on the application of tilt, recline, and elevating legrests for wheelchairs literature update. *Assist Technol.* 2015;27(3):193–198. https://doi.org/10.1080/10400435.2015.1066657

Dicianno BE, Schmeler M, Liu B. Wheelchairs/adaptive mobility equipment and seating. In: Campagnolo DI, Kirshblum S, Nash MS, et al., eds. *Spinal Cord Medicine.* 2nd ed. Lippincott Williams & Wilkins; 2012:341–358.

A 78-year-old, right-handed man with a right middle cerebral artery stroke and left hemiparesis presents for an assistive technology evaluation in an outpatient clinic. He completed inpatient and outpatient rehabilitation but has not regained ambulation ability that is sufficient enough for him to be able to complete activities of daily living inside the home, and he is not able to go out into the community due to fear of falling.

Questions

1. What key elements about his history would you need to elicit?

2. What aspects of the physical exam will you collect? Explain why you will collect each component of the exam.

He was discharged from inpatient rehabilitation with a rented folding light-weight manual wheelchair with adjustable tension backrest, standard foam cushion, and removable leg rests. He cannot push it because of his hemiparesis. He uses a wheeled walker and an ankle-foot orthosis (AFO) when he ambulates. He can ambulate and transfer independently but describes his walking as slow. He denies significant spasticity or falls. He has some mild left shoulder pain but it does not limit his activity. He does not have a wheelchair of his own. He wants a device that is easily transportable. He lives with his wife who has back pain, and they have a small compact car. He is retired and wants to spend time with his grandchildren. They live in a very small apartment that has two steps to enter and cannot be ramped.

On exam, he has normal strength in the right hemi-body. He has no pain with testing of the left shoulder, and deltoids are 2/5. Distally, his strength is 3/5 in the arm. In the left lower limb, hip flexors are 2/5, quadriceps 3/5, hip adductors 4/5, and dorsiflexors 2/5. Sensation is decreased on the left hemi-body but normal on the right. Tone is Modified Ashworth Scale 2 in the left arm and leg. Range of motion is normal, but his left shoulder is slightly subluxed. There is a mild left visual neglect. Transfers are modified independent with a walker. Gait is functionally slow and hemiparetic with impaired swing of the left leg. The leg is slightly externally rotated when he advances it.

3. Why is the patient displaying this particular gait impairment despite using a brace?

4. What assistive technology intervention would be indicated for this patient?

During a trial in clinic, the patient is able to propel an ultralight manual wheelchair with his arms but using one leg does improve maneuverability. You notice that he is having trouble grasping the push rim because of spasticity in his fingers.

5. What interventions could you suggest to improve his grasp?

The patient is concerned about insurance coverage for a wheelchair. He has Medicare.

6. How might you address his question about insurance coverage of a wheelchair?

He asks whether wheelchair propulsion can increase shoulder pain.

7. What education should be provided to this patient?

Answers

1. Obtain information about the type of assistive technology that he has used so far (e.g., wheelchair, assistive device such as a cane or crutch, orthoses). Ask about level of independence with transfers and ambulation. Obtain review of systems data regarding spasticity, falls, and pain. Obtain information about what type of technology he would like, employment status, and social history, including his mode of transportation.

2. Evaluate strength, muscle tone, sensation, range of motion, and transfers to assess how these factors may be influencing his gait. Also evaluate for any visual neglect that could impact his gait or use of a mobility device. Perform a thorough musculoskeletal examination of the shoulder to determine if he will have problems propelling a wheelchair or using an assistive device.

3. Although the patient's foot drop is corrected with the brace, the patient has weak hip flexors that are causing problems advancing the leg. He is using the stronger hip adductors to advance the leg. Additionally, spasticity, decreased sensation, and neglect may be contributing to impaired functional mobility.

4. One choice for this patient would be an ultralight manual wheelchair. A low seat height would allow him to propel with one arm and one leg. A manual wheelchair could be used both inside and outside the apartment, but his wife would likely need to assist with getting the wheelchair up and down the steps and into the vehicle. A power wheelchair would not be able to be used inside and outside unless the entrance was ramped. A small scooter could possibly be disassembled and reassembled to get it into and out of the home or the trunk of a car, but that may be too cumbersome for his wife, and the turning radius of a scooter may preclude its use in small areas in the apartment.

5. The patient may be a candidate for management of his spasticity, with consideration of targeted treatment of finger flexors with botulinum toxin, if the goal is to improve functional grasp. A specialized push rim that is coated or has an ergonomic shape may also facilitate propulsion. Wheelchair propulsion training is also indicated.

6. Medicare Part B covers 80% of durable medical equipment such as wheelchairs.

7. Explain that the wheelchair needs to be custom fit and configured and that optimal axle position is important for shoulder health. He requires education on wheelchair skills and propulsion patterns, wheelchair maintenance, and joint preservation. Explain that low seat height will allow for some propulsion one leg. Follow-up with physiatry will be needed if shoulder pain worsens or for ongoing treatment of spasticity.

BIBLIOGRAPHY

Cooper RA. Manual wheelchairs. In: Cooper RA, ed. *Wheelchair Selection and Configuration*. Demos Medical Publishing;1998:199–223.

Medicare. Durable medical equipment coverage. https://www.medicare.gov/coverage/durable-medical-equipment-coverage.html

An 82-year-old female with end-stage right hip osteoarthritis presents to your outpatient clinic due to falls. She complains of right hip pain and tells you that she has not been interested in hip surgery due to her age and other comorbid conditions, including a prior myocardial infarction. She would like to know what she can do to prevent falls. She describes her balance as poor.

Questions

1. What key elements about her history would you need to elicit?

2. What aspects of the physical exam will you collect? Explain why you will collect each component of the exam.

She describes her falls as being accompanied by pain and her hip "giving out." She denies loss of consciousness or tripping over objects. She uses a cane. She is right-handed and prefers using the cane in that hand. She recently finished physical therapy but is still having pain and occasionally falling. Her medication list includes aspirin, a beta-blocker, an antianxiety medication (lorazepam), and an anticholinergic medication for her bladder, but she says that she does not like to take medications and takes only acetaminophen. She denies any diabetes or loss of sensation. She recently had cataract surgery and describes her vision as "good." She is not interested in any type of wheeled mobility device. On exam, she has 4+ to 5/5 strength in the lower body, except for the right hip. Although pain-inhibited, her strength in the right hip abductors and flexors is 4-. Sensation and muscle bulk are normal. Passive range of motion of her right hip is limited by pain, but her left hip range of motion is normal. During stance phase on the right, the left side of her pelvis tilts down and her trunk leans to the right. Her gait is also antalgic on the right. Her elbow is flexed approximately 25 degrees when using the cane. Explain why the patient is perceiving balance problems.

3. Why is the patient displaying this particular gait impairment?

4. What intervention would be indicated for this patient?

The patient says that she enjoyed physical therapy, but it was painful and she is not sure whether her hip strength got any better as a result.

5. What interventions could you suggest to improve hip strength?

You decide to implement a screening process for falls in your clinic.

6. How might you begin to implement such a program?

She is reluctant to use a walker due to cosmetic considerations.

7. How would you counsel her?

Answers

1. Obtain information about the nature of her falls (e.g., mechanical, syncope). Ask about assistive device use and assess whether the devices have been used properly. Enquire about any therapies received. Evaluate for other etiologies for falling, such as multiple medication usage, low vision, or peripheral neuropathy.

2. Evaluate strength, muscle bulk, sensation, range of motion, and gait. Also evaluate for any visual impairments. Perform a thorough musculoskeletal examination of the hip.

3. The patient has a compensated Trendelenburg gait because of right hip abductor weakness. She is compensating for the drop in her pelvis with a trunk lean to the right. The antalgic gait on the right causes her to spend less time in stance phase on the right. Because she is using a cane on the antalgic side, she is also loading her right hip with unnecessary force during walking.

4. The cane seems to be at the proper height since the elbow is flexed between 20 and 30 degrees, but should be switched to the left side to offload the right hip during ambulation. Physical therapy may be required to train her to use the cane properly or to trial a walker.

5. Isometric resistance strength training is generally indicated in the presence of a painful joint because it is better tolerated from a pain perspective. Aquatic therapy can also be beneficial in the setting of osteoarthritis because the buoyancy of the water helps offload painful joints and allows the patient to exhibit greater range of motion, with the water providing some resistance.

6. Consider using a validated fall risk survey. To be cost- and time-effective, a questionnaire could be completed while the patient is in the waiting area or with assistance from staff. A physical or occupational therapist could also administer a functional evaluation to screen for falls in the clinic or conduct a home safety evaluation. You may consider carrying out a quality improvement project to determine whether your screening is effective by following up with patients over time.

7. Be sensitive to her concerns and acknowledge them. Discuss adapting to disability and how assistive technology can improve function and preserve independence. Remind her of the risks of falling, and how a hip fracture or other injuries might impact her. Discuss the risks and benefits of using different assistive technologies and encourage her to make an educated choice. The discussion may need to continue in future visits.

BIBLIOGRAPHY

Bennell KL, Dobson F, Hinman RS. Exercise in osteoarthritis: moving from prescription to adherence. *Best Pract Res Clin Rheumatol.* 2014;28(1):93–117. https://doi.org/10.1016/j.berh.2014.01.009

Blount WP. Don't throw away the cane. *J Bone Joint Surg Am.* 1956;38-A(3):695–708. https://doi.org/10.2106/00004623-195638030-00023

Kumar R, Roe MC, Scremin OU. Methods for estimating the proper length of a cane. *Arch Phys Med Rehabil.* 1995;76(12):1173–1175. https://doi.org/10.1016/S0003-9993(95)80129-4

A 22-year-old male with T9 AIS A spinal cord injury presents to your assistive technology outpatient clinic for a mobility device evaluation. His current manual wheelchair is in disrepair and he is interested in a wheelchair he saw on a website.

Questions

1. What key elements about his history would you need to elicit?

2. What aspects of the physical exam will you collect? Explain why you will collect each component of the exam.

He currently uses a folding (cross-brace) manual wheelchair that is about 5 years old. He is able to transfer independently. He is employed as an accountant and drives an adapted vehicle. He wants to start playing wheelchair basketball and tennis. He has a prior rotator cuff tear that was repaired, but he has some residual right shoulder pain that does not limit activity. He has a remote history of a pressure injury on his sacrum but no recent skin breakdown. He is mostly continent of bowel and bladder when compliant with his bladder and bowel routines. On exam, he has 5/5 strength in the upper body and 0/5 strength in the lower body. He has increased tone in the legs. Sensory level is at T9. Trunk balance is fair. Contractures are noted at the knees, but passive shoulder range of motion is normal. His right shoulder exam is relatively normal. Skin is intact.

3. Explain how choosing a wheelchair and setting it up properly can help to mitigate shoulder pain.

4. The patient asks you to explain the advantages of solid frame ultra-light wheelchairs compared to folding frames.

You order an ultralight manual wheelchair with a customizable axle.

5. What effect does fore/aft axle position have on wheelchair propulsion?

This patient wants to participate in two different adaptive sports, basketball and tennis.

6. Explain what technology he would need and how it might be funded.

This patient wants to know how he can help himself continue to be athletic and independent as he ages.

7. How might you counsel this patient?

Answers

1. Obtain information about his current wheelchair, including frame type. Obtain a functional history to include transfer ability. Ask about social history, including employment, transportation, and leisure activities. Conduct a thorough review of systems, including history of shoulder pain, incontinence, and skin breakdown.

2. Evaluate strength, muscle tone, trunk balance, sensation, and range of motion to understand his positioning needs. Evaluate transfer ability. Inspect skin for breakdown. Perform a thorough musculoskeletal examination of the shoulder to determine whether he has issues with wheelchair propulsion.

3. Keeping the weight of the individual and the wheelchair minimized, teaching proper wheelchair propulsion technique, and proper setup of the wheelchair (including axle position) can help to mitigate shoulder pain.

4. Solid frames are available as cantilever or box designs. Because they are solid, efficiency of propulsion and durability are higher than with a folding frame. Although the frames do not fold, they have quick-release wheels and the backrests can be folded down for ease of transportability.

5. A rearward axle reduces access to the push rim, promoting an "arc" style of propulsion and increasing the strokes required to travel a given distance, and thereby predisposing the user to repetitive strain injuries. A rearward axle also makes the chair more stable. A forward axle promotes propulsion using long, smooth strokes (semicircular pattern), reducing stroke frequency. Moving the axle forward allows the chair to tip backward more easily for wheelies but moving it too far forward can make the chair unstable.

6. A person's everyday wheelchair is not typically used for sports. Each sport has its own wheelchair design that is geared specifically for that sport. Ideally, this person would need to use both basketball and tennis wheelchairs. However, sports equipment is not covered under standard private medical insurance. (Some options, however, are available for those with Veterans Affairs coverage.) Typically, individuals would need to self-pay or identify other private funding sources if they wanted their own sports equipment. However, it would be helpful to refer this patient to a local adaptive sports organization that can get him started in sports and that may have equipment that participants share.

7. Explain that assistive technology can promote functional independence for activities of daily living, community integration, and physical activities, including sports. Explain that often, technology needs to be custom-fit and configured for optimal function, and that regular repair and maintenance will be needed. Discuss the fact that technology is always advancing so regular follow-up may be needed, especially as his needs change. Reinforce the

importance of preservation of the shoulder, which depends on a number of factors, including his ability maintain a healthy weight and propel with proper form. Explain that shoulder health will also help maintain his ability to transfer. Explain that preventive care is important for long-term health in spinal cord injury, especially prevention of pressure injuries.

BIBLIOGRAPHY

Cooper RA. Sports and alternative wheelchairs. In: Cooper RA, ed. *Wheelchair Selection and Configuration.* Demos Medical Publishing; 1998:271–290.

Dicianno B, Schmeler M, Liu B. Wheelchairs/adaptive mobility equipment and seating. In: Campagnolo DI, Kirshblum S, Nash MS, et al., eds. *Spinal Cord Medicine.* 2nd ed. Lippincott Williams & Wilkins; 2012:341–358 [VN12].

A 52-year-old female with multiple sclerosis, diagnosed 6 months ago, presents to your assistive technology outpatient clinic for a mobility device evaluation. She has been using a depot (standard) manual wheelchair that she self-purchased, but she is having trouble propelling it because it is heavy and because of upper limb weakness and fatigue. She is looking for a device to improve her mobility indoors and outdoors.

Questions

1. What key elements about her history would you need to elicit?

2. What aspects of the physical exam will you collect? Explain why you will collect each component of the exam.

She is able to walk independently with a left AFO and a walker but gets fatigued after only a couple steps, which sometimes results in falls. She worked as a nurse's aide but is now unemployed. She would like to seek a different job. She was driving a compact car but stopped due to leg weakness. She enjoys traveling to visit her adult children and cooking. She lives with her husband in a small condominium. She has diffuse muscle cramps and admits to having a difficult time dealing with her diagnosis. On exam, she has 4/5 strength in the upper body, 2/5 strength in the left hip flexor and dorsiflexors, and 4/5 strength in the lower body otherwise. Tone is normal. Trunk balance is fair. Range of motion is normal. She needed assistance from her husband to transfer out of the wheelchair.

3. Explain why the patient's transfer ability is important to consider when choosing a mobility device.

4. The patient asks about a scooter because she has used them in the past in the grocery store. What are the pros and cons of a scooter, compared to a power wheelchair, for this particular patient?

The patient asks how she could use the power seat functions on a power wheelchair to prevent skin breakdown.

5. Explain how you could use these features to offload pressure and address skin breakdown.

This patient again brings up that finding a new job is important to her, and the fact that this may involve figuring out how to transport a wheelchair.

6. What counseling would you give her, and what other referrals might be indicated for this patient?

She is distraught about her progressive disability. She becomes tearful over the fact that she now needs a power wheelchair.

7. How might you counsel this patient?

Answers

1. Obtain information about her ability to walk and transfer, as well as assistive device use. Ask about social history, including employment, living environment, transportation, and leisure activities. Conduct a thorough review of systems, including history of pain and depressive symptoms.

2. Conduct a musculoskeletal and neurologic exam to include strength, muscle tone, trunk balance, and range of motion to understand her seating and positioning needs. Assess her ability to transfer.

3. If a person cannot transfer or weight shift independently, the person may be at risk for skin breakdown, and therefore may need a device with power seat functions that allows the patient to reposition independently.

4. Scooters (Figure 6.1) are sometimes viewed by patients more favorably because they are familiar from retail environments. Scooters are less expensive than power wheelchairs. However, scooters have a wide turning radius that makes them less maneuverable in tight living spaces, can tip over on uneven surfaces, and require more shoulder function to operate since they have a tiller. They also have no power features that assist weight shifting. A power wheelchair with power seat functions may therefore be the better option for this patient.

5. Power tilt allows a patient to change their seat angle orientation in relation to the ground while maintaining a constant seat-to-back angle and seat-to-leg-rest angle. This allows a user to transfer pressure from the ischial tuberosities to the sacrum and back. Power recline allows a patient to increase their seat-to-back angle, which lies them more supine and spreads pressure over more surface area. Recline can cause shear on the skin when used alone. Typically, a combination of tilt and recline used together can offload the most pressure from the ischial tuberosities.

6. If she transitions to using a power wheelchair, she will need to explore different options for transporting the wheelchair, including an accessible van with a lift or public transportation. Vehicles and vehicle modifications are not covered by most commercial medical insurers. Accessible shuttle transportation may be an option for medical visits but is not available in many rural areas. This patient may benefit from being referred to vocational rehabilitation or a rehabilitation counselor given her interest in seeking a different job and considerations for transportation costs related to employment. Also consider referral to an adaptive driving program for driving training and recommendations on transportation options.

7. Acknowledge that multiple sclerosis can be particularly frustrating due to the unpredictability of prognosis. Most patients do well and have slow progression, but some patients have more difficulty. Offer psychological consultation, referral for spiritual or religious guidance, and/or referral to patient support groups, many of which are available online.

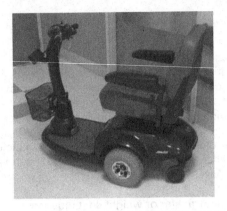

Figure 6.1 Power scooter.

BIBLIOGRAPHY

Cooper RA. Manual wheelchairs. In: Cooper RA, ed. *Wheelchair Selection and Configuration*. Demos Medical Publishing; 1998:199–223.

Dicianno BE, Lieberman J, Schmeler MR, et al. Rehabilitation engineering and assistive technology society of North America's position on the application of tilt, recline, and elevating legrests for wheelchairs literature update. *Assist Technol*. 2015;27(3):193–198. https://doi.org/10.1080/10400435.2015.1066657

An 18-year-old female with spastic quadriplegic cerebral palsy presents to your outpatient assistive technology clinic because of problems with her power wheelchair. She is accompanied by her parents. She has severe dysarthria, and her parents communicate most of the information to you.

Questions

1. What key elements about her history would you need to elicit?

2. What aspects of the physical exam will you collect? Explain why you will collect each component of the exam.

The wheelchair has a problem with the brakes and is about 1 year old. It has a pressure relief cushion and power seat functions including tilt, recline, and elevating leg rests. She is able to operate the joystick and controls for power seat functions. Her parents do most of the talking, although the patient tries to interject occasionally. Her parents say that they understand her speech and will finish her sentences for her, and they do this because it is faster to communicate that way. On exam, she is not able to transfer independently and has poor trunk control. She has antigravity strength in the upper body and less than gravity strength in the lower body. Manual muscle testing is difficult to assess because of diffuse spasticity and contractures, and involuntary synergistic movement in the legs. The patient seems frustrated. Her speech is severely dysarthric. She can control all aspects of her power wheelchair.

3. What assistive technology interventions might be appropriate for her?

4. Discuss how you would explain to the patient and family the concept of an augmentative and alternative communication (AAC) device.

5. Explain how an AAC device can assist users with different types of disabilities affecting speech and language.

The patient seems excited about the possibility of using an AAC device and wants to know how she can be evaluated and whether her insurance will cover this.

6. What type of referral and advice would you provide to her?

Because the patient is frustrated with her family talking over her, you want to improve the patient's and family's communication during the visit.

7. Before she receives an AAC device, what strategies could you use to improve communication?

Answers

1. Obtain information about the problems she is having with her power wheelchair and its age and features. Ask about the communication strategies that the patient uses with others.

2. Conduct a musculoskeletal and neurologic exam to include strength, muscle tone, trunk balance, and range of motion to understand her seating and positioning needs. Assess her ability to transfer. Inspect the skin for breakdown. Inspect the wheelchair seating configuration and features. Assess her speech and language.

3. Given the age of the power wheelchair, brake repair (rather than a new wheelchair) is likely indicated. Most importantly, however, the patient may also benefit from an AAC device to assist with communication.

4. AAC devices can augment or assist communication by providing a platform for users to select information they want to convey. AAC devices may be high-tech or low-tech, and include word boards, communication books, electronic tablet speech applications, and speech-generating devices.

5. Dysarthria occurs when there is an impairment of motor control of speech resulting in incoordination, weakness, or slowing of speech. Apraxia occurs when there is an impairment of coordination of peripheral muscles, such as those used for writing. Aphasia occurs when comprehension, fluency, repetition, or naming is impaired. AAC systems can be used to assist or augment communication when any of these impairments occur.

6. Refer her to a speech language pathologist with experience with AAC device evaluations. Most commercial medical insurances cover AAC devices in general, but some insurers cover specific makes or models of devices or software. It would also be important to consult with the rehabilitation engineer, wheelchair supplier, and/or therapist involved in providing the wheelchair because an AAC device can be mounted on and draw power from the wheelchair itself.

7. Speak directly to the patient and look at her when you communicate. Provide her ample time to communicate her thoughts. Ask her to repeat anything that you do not understand. Provide her time to speak with you privately, without the parents in the room, if she wishes. Acknowledge the input of the family as important in the decision-making process, but also reinforce the fact that you want to hear the thoughts and opinion of the patient in her own words and want to give her the ability to make educated choices.

BIBLIOGRAPHY

Assistive Technologies: Principles and Practice. By Albert M. Cook PhD PE (ret.) and Janice Miller Polgar BScOT PhD FCAOT. January 1, 2015; Mosby, 4th edition.

7 Geriatric Rehabilitation

George Forrest

An 80-year-old man is admitted to the hospital with community-acquired pneumonia. He is treated with ceftriaxone and azithromycin. On the eighth day of admission, the hospitalist tells the patient that he has completed his course of antibiotics and he can go home. The patient tells the doctor, "I do not think I am ready to go home. I feel very weak. I do not think that I can climb the stairs at the entrance to my home, and I would not feel safe getting into and out of my tub." You are asked to evaluate the patient.

Questions

1. What would be important parts of the history that you obtain from the patient and from the patient's medical record?

The patient tells you that before he was admitted to the hospital he considered his health to be good for his age. He is living at home with his wife, who is 78, and they had no help other than a woman who comes to help with cleaning once a week. He was not intubated or treated with steroids. He feels generally weak but he does not notice focal weakness or numbness.

2. What would be important parts of the physical examination?

The patient's vital signs are normal. There is no drop in blood pressure when going from supine to sit. The heart is regular, the lungs are clear, the abdomen is benign, and there is no edema. The patient is alert and oriented. His responses to questions are all given with good logic and detail. His cranial nerve examination is normal. Reflexes are normal throughout all extremities. There is no alteration in tone or cogwheel rigidity. The patient moves all extremities through a full range of motion against gravity. You can very easily break his strength when he tries to maintain elevation of his shoulders. He has difficulty coming from sit to stand without rocking back and forth and pushing off with both hands.

3. What likely has happened to impair this patient's transfers and function?

The patient tells you that he has been in the hospital for a week. During that time he did not feel well, so he really got out of bed only to go to the bathroom.

4. What are some of the physiologic changes that occur in patients who are at bed rest for a week?

5. What can be done to treat his weakness?

6. Describe elements of a quality improvement to engage staff on the acute medical unit to mobilize patients early in their hospital stay.

The patient is reluctant to get out of bed. He says he is tired, and he never exercises much at home.

7. How can you motivate him to engage in mobility?

Answers

1. You would want to know the patient's level of function prior to admission. You would want to know if the patient was intubated, was treated with steroids, had positive blood cultures, or multi-organ failure, as these factors are associated with critical illness neuropathy/myopathy. You would want to know if the patient had any symptoms of a focal neurologic process such has a hemiplegia, sensory deficit, or focal weakness. You should ask about his home situation, including environmental barriers and family support.

2. You would want to check the vital signs in particular, making sure that the fever has resolved and that the patient does not have orthostatic hypotension. You want to do a careful neurologic examination to make sure that there is no evidence of underlying Parkinson's disease, dementia, stroke, spinal cord injury, cerebellar disease, peroneal nerve injury, radiculopathy, or peripheral neuropathy. You should observe the patient doing bed mobility, transfers, and gait.

3. There are many possible causes of weakness in this patient. The list would include inflammatory muscle disease, connective tissue disease, vasculitis, hypothyroid or hyperthyroid disease, viral myositis, rhabdomyolysis, neuromuscular junction disease, paraneoplastic syndrome, hypokalemia, hypophosphatemia, low magnesium level, medications, demyelinating disease, radiculopathy, or medications. The history and examination do not suggest any of these problems. The most likely cause is weakness related to prolonged bedrest.

4. Muscle strength may decline by 1% to 1.5% per day. Antigravity muscles of lower extremities are affected more than muscles of the upper extremities. Patients on bed rest lose 1% of bone mass of the vertebrae per week of bed rest. Patients on bed rest have a decrease in plasma volume. This results in increased heart rate at rest and with activity, decreased stroke volume, and orthostatic hypotension. Bed rest is associated with coagulopathy and increased risk of venous thrombosis. Bed rest is associated with increased insulin resistance and glucose intolerance and with atelectasis, impaired respiratory function, and predisposition to pneumonia.

5. Studies show that giving patients exercises to do in bed, encouraging patients to get out of bed, and providing active therapies prevent the development of disuse atrophy. Simple bed-based exercises with elastic bands and pedal cycles can start. Getting the patient up to a chair a few hours a day, and short walks if feasible, can make a tremendous impact.

6. Start by forming an interprofessional team with internal medicine, nursing, physical therapy (PT), and occupational therapy (OT). Engage them with data showing the deleterious effects of bed rest. Start tracking the functional status and activity level of patients with validated tools. Engage nursing and

therapies to work together to mobilize patients, with nursing being the primary driving force for more easily mobilized patients without neurologic or musculoskeletal impairments and therapies to mobilize more complex patients.

7. Use motivational interviewing techniques to identify the patient's perceived barriers to mobility and addressing those. Is pain an issue? Are there reversible causes for fatigue? Have the patient identify benefits of increased mobility on his quality of life.

BIBLIOGRAPHY

Hoyer EH, Friedman M, Lavezza A, et al. Promoting mobility and reducing LOS. *J Hosp Med.* 2016;5:341–347. https://doi.org/10.1002/jhm.2546

Parry SM, Putcheary ZA. The impact of extended bed rest on the musculoskeletal system in the critical care environment. *Extrem Physiol Med.* 2015;4:16. https://doi.org/10.1186/s13728-015-0036-7

Saguil A. Evaluation of the patient with muscle weakness. *Am Fam Physician.* 2005;71(7):1327–1336.

Topp R, Ditmyer M, King K, et al. The effect of bed rest and the potential of prehabilitation on patients in the intensive care unit. *AACN Clin Issues.* 2002;13(2):263–276. https://doi.org/10.1097/00044067-200205000-00011

CASE 2

A 67-year-old woman comes to your office. She tells you that her joints hurt. Her left knee is swollen and she has pain when she walks.

Questions

1. What more do you want to know about the patient's history, comorbidities, and social situation?

The patient has insidious onset of pain, mostly affecting her left knee. Pain hurts mostly with standing and walking. She has trouble climbing her stairs.

2. How would you go about performing physical examination of this patient?

She is afebrile. The patient has a left knee valgus deformity. She has a small effusion of left knee. There is no instability, warmth, or erythema. Range of motion is 0 to 95 degrees. She has bony overgrowth of the distal interphalangeal joints of fingers two to four both hands. Other joints are normal. Gait is antalgic to the left.

3. What is the differential diagnosis of this patient?

4. What diagnostic tests would you perform?

Laboratory tests are normal. The x-ray of the left knee shows bony proliferation and osteophytes at the margins of the joint, asymmetrical narrowing of the joint space, and subchondral cysts. There is a calcified loose body in the joint. Joint fluid gram stain and examination for crystals are negative.

5. Outline a treatment plan.

The patient tells you that she has a high deductible and high co-pay insurance plan. She cannot afford PT.

6. What suggestions do you have?

The patient tells you that her sister just had a knee replacement. She wants to know if this is an option for her.

7. How would you explain to her indications, risks, and benefits of this surgery?

Answers

1. Duration of pain and swelling? Which joints hurt? What time of the day the joints hurt and for how long they hurt? What activities are associated with increased pain and which with relief of pain? Has there been trauma? Fever or chills? How does the pain limit your function? Does she have environmental barriers, such as stairs? You are interested in whether she might have inflammatory or traumatic arthritis. You want to know the impact on her activities of daily living (ADLs).

2. Check vital signs looking for fever. Do a detailed musculoskeletal examination looking for evidence of synovitis or tender joints. Observe the knees for valgus or varus deformity. Check the left knee for effusion, stability, warmth, tenderness, and erythema. Record range of motion and feel for crepitance. Check drawer sign, Apley's compression/distraction. Observe the skin for stigmata of systemic disease such as psoriatic lesions, gouty tophi, rheumatoid nodules. Watch the patient walk. You are looking for systemic disease. You are looking for signs of osteoarthritis.

3. The distribution of joints involved is consistent with osteoarthritis. The patient has Heberden nodes and Bouchard nodes and involvement of at least one large joint. The distribution of lesions is not suggestive of rheumatoid arthritis. The patient does not have the systemic symptoms of systemic lupus erythematosus (SLE). The patient could have superimposed gout, pseudo-gout, or infection.

4. Check x-ray of the knee and do a complete blood count (CBC), rheumatoid factor, C-reactive protein (CRP) or erythrocyte sedimentation rate (ESR), and uric acid. If the effusion is large, consider aspirating the joint for crystal analysis and cell counts.

5. The x-rays and laboratory studies confirm a diagnosis of osteoarthritis. Options for immediate pain control are nonsteroidal anti-inflammatory drug (NSAID) medication or local injection. An injection of corticosteroid into the affected knee can provide temporary relief of pain. There is a very small risk of infection. The steroid may accelerate deterioration of the cartilage and cause weakening of ligaments, so it should not be done more than two to three times per year. Nonsteroidal anti-inflammatory agents are more effective than acetaminophen but they are associated with gastrointestinal bleeding, renal insufficiency, fluid retention, hypertension, congestive heart failure, and possibly coronary artery disease. They should be used judiciously in patients taking angiotensin inhibitors, angiotensin receptor blockers, or anticoagulants. Capsaicin crème or topical anti-inflammatory agents may help. There are studies showing that duloxetine is helpful. A cane in the contralateral hand may reduce pain. Weight loss is helpful for patients with increased body mass index. PT is helpful. Therapy may include stretching to relieve tightness of the hip flexors, adductors and abductors, quadriceps muscle, hamstrings,

and gastrocnemius muscles. Strengthening of the hip extensors, hamstrings, and quadriceps is important. Exercises that do not stress the swollen knee joint include isometric quadriceps sets, terminal knee extension, straight leg raising, bicycle with raised seat height, and pool therapy. There are studies that suggest that injection with platelet-rich plasma is helpful, but at this time, the strength of evidence is not rated as high. There is not sufficient data to determine if knee braces are helpful. Treatments to avoid are glucosamine chondroitin sulfate, injection with hyaluronic acid, wash out of the knee, and prescription of heel wedges. Arthroscopic debridement or repair of torn meniscus is not helpful.

6. You can prepare written handouts with exercise programs for your patients. You can refer the patient to exercise programs available through any search engine. You can advise on exercise programs available on YouTube and programs at organizations such as the Young Men's Christian Association (YMCA).

7. Tell her that this is a very well-established operation. Seventy percent to 90% of patients have improvement in pain and function. The rates of infection and complication of thrombosis are low when the procedure is done by skilled surgeons. The prosthesis can be expected to last 15 years. It is major surgery with a relatively long recovery measured in months to a year. Recommend a trial of conservative therapy. Indications for surgery are poorly controlled pain and limitations in function, work, recreation, and quality of life that are not acceptable to the patient.

BIBLIOGRAPHY

Choosing Wisely American Academy of Orthopedic Surgeons. https://www.choosingwisely.org/societies/american-academy-of-orthopaedic-surgeons/#:~:text=The%20American%20Academy%20of%20Orthopaedic,of%20bone%20and%20joint%20health

Ebell MH. Osteoarthritis: rapid evidence review. *Am Fam Physician.* 2018;97(8):524–526.

Lin KW. Treatment of knee osteoarthritis. *Am Fam Physician.* 2018;98(9):602–606.

Vakharia RM, Roche MW, Alcerro JC, et al. The current status of cell-based therapies for primary knee osteoarthritis. *Orthop Clin North Am.* 2019;50(4):415–423. https://doi.org/10.1016/j.ocl.2019.06.001

A 75-year-old lady comes to the office with her daughter. The daughter tells you that she is worried about her mom. "Mom feels well. She never complains but she just doesn't look steady on her feet. I am afraid she is going to fall."

Questions

1. What questions would you ask the patient?

The patient tells you that she has noticed that her gait is slower. She has not fallen but she just does not feel as steady as she used to. She is not sure why. She feels well. She does not take any medicines except for atorvastatin and amlodipine. She never feels like she is going to blackout and never has any sense of dizziness or spinning. She does not feel weak and has no numbness. Her friends all have problems with their backs or joints but she is lucky she does not have those problems.

2. Describe the key portions of your examination.

The patient's vital signs are normal and there is no orthostatic hypotension. Examination of the heart lungs abdomen and extremities are normal. Score on the Mini-Mental State Examination is 30. The patient's vision is 20/30. She has some trouble hearing you when you whisper. Tone, reflexes, and manual muscle tests are normal. The patient has no difficulty distinguishing sharp from dull, but proprioception seems mildly impaired. The patient can feel the vibration of a tuning fork placed on the patella but not on the medial malleolus or the first toe (bilaterally). There is no past pointing, and alternating movements do not show dysdiadochokinesia. The patient's gait has a normal heel-to-toe pattern and appears stable, but the Romberg's test shows some sway when standing with the eyes closed.

3. What special tests could you do in the office or ask the physical therapist to perform to help assess the risk that the patient might fall?

4. What do you think is wrong with the patient? What laboratory and diagnostic tests might you request?

5. What interventions could reduce the risk of falls?

Her daughter thinks it would be a good idea for her mother to have a home health aide.

6. The daughter asks if Medicare will cover this expense. How should you respond?

The patient gets angry at her daughter during the visit. "Stop answering questions for me." She also feels her daughter is being overprotective.

7. How would you mediate this dispute?

Answers

1. Ask the patient if she has fallen or if she is afraid of falling or if she has noticed a change in her gait. Obtain a full history of her medical problems. Ask which medications she takes. Obtain a full review of systems in particular, wanting to know if there are symptoms of dizziness at rest, with change in position, or when going from supine to sit or sit to stand. Ask if the patient has palpitations or a history of arrhythmias. Inquire about change in vision, hearing, or tinnitus. Determine if there was a history of focal weakness or numbness or if the patient noted any change in muscle tone, strength, or balance. Find out if she had any painful conditions suggestive of radiculopathy or problems with her joints or her feet.

2. Check vital signs including a check for orthostatic hypotension. Listen to her heart checking for arrhythmia. You evaluate her joints and spine for range of and examine her feet. Perform a cognitive evaluation such as the Mini-Mental State Exam or the Montreal Cognitive Assessment Test. Check the patient's vision with an eye card. Evaluate hearing by the patient's ability to hear a whispered voice, watch, or tuning fork at about 2 feet from the ear. Examine the patient's tone looking for rigidity or cog wheeling. Check reflexes and perform a manual muscle test of all four extremities. Evaluate appreciation of light touch, pinprick proprioception, and vibration. Have the patient perform finger-nose-finger, alternating hand movements, and heel-to-shin testing. Have the patient do a Romberg's test and watch the patient walk.

3. Two tests that can easily be performed in the office are the timed up and go (TUG) test and the functional reach test. In the TUG test, the patient is asked to get up from a chair, walk 3 m, and walk back to the chair and sit down. Ten seconds is considered a normal time and patients with a time of more than 14 seconds are considered at risk of fall. In the functional reach test, the patient stands with their feet shoulder-width apart. The patient raises one arm to 90 degrees of flexion and is asked to reach forward without taking a step. Most patients can extend the third metacarpal at least 10 inches forward. A score of 6 to 7 inches is considered indicative of impaired balance. The Berg balance test is more time consuming. The patient is asked to perform 14 different maneuvers and each one is graded 0 to 4. The maneuvers are:

Sit to stand	standing to sitting	placing a foot on a stool
Stand unsupported	reaching forward	standing one foot in front of other
Sit unsupported	retrieving object from floor	standing on one foot
Standing with eyes closes	looking over shoulder	transfer chair to chair
Standing with feet together	turning 360 degrees	

A score of more than 40 is considered a low risk of fall. Twenty-one to 40 is a moderate risk of fall and 0 to 20 is a high risk for fall.

4. The history and examination do not suggest a problem with the heart or orthostasis. There are no symptoms or signs of vestibular disease, arthritis, or other musculoskeletal problem. There is no indication of stroke, myelopathy, myopathy, or Parkinson's disease. The most common reason that a 70-year-old person would have difficulty with gait is age-related decline in the function of three systems involved with regulation of balance. These are the vestibular, vision, and proprioception systems. The patient has impaired proprioception and appreciation of vibration and a positive Romberg's test. An electromyography (EMG)/nerve conduction velocity (NCV) test to evaluate for peripheral neuropathy would be helpful. A basic set of laboratory studies to investigate for peripheral neuropathy might include hemoglobin A1C, chemistry profile including fasting blood sugar, creatinine, and liver function tests. Vitamin B12, thyroid function tests, ESR serum protein electrophoresis (SPEP), and antinuclear antibody (ANA). Albumin can help assess nutritional status. Vitamin D deficiency is associated with muscle weakness and increased risk of fall. Additional tests that might be ordered in some patients depending upon the history include HIV serology, rheumatoid factor, Sjogren's syndrome testing (anti-Ro, anti-La antibodies), anti-Lyme antibodies, Vitamin B1, and hepatitis panel. This patient takes atorvastatin so a creatine phosphokinase (CPK) might be helpful.

5. Studies have shown that exercise programs to improve strength, balance, and endurance can reduce the rate of falls. Recommendations for home safety include making sure that there is proper lighting and that there are railings on all staircases. Walking surfaces should provide good footing (eliminate shag rugs, throw rugs, electrical cords, and clutter). Grab-bars and handrails should be installed in the bathroom to increase safety during toileting and washing. The kitchen and bedrooms should be arranged to minimize the need for reaching and climbing.

6. Unfortunately, Medicare will only cover a home health aide for a few hours a week and only while the patient is also receiving skilled home care visits (RN, PT, OT, and/or speech-language pathology [SLP]). Hiring home health aides can be very expensive—$200 to $300/day. A less expensive alternative may be an electronic alert system worn as a necklace or bracelet.

7. Explain to the daughter that you really need to hear directly from the patient about her concerns. At the same time, reassure the patient that her daughter is concerned about her and is expressing some important concerns.

BIBLIOGRAPHY

Forrest G, Schott Z, Radu G. Geriatric gait and balance disorders. mc.aapmr/kn/article.html?id=79
Salzman B. Gait and balance disorders in older adults. Am Fam Physician. 2010;82:61–68.
Snijders AH, Van de Warrenburg BP, Giladi N, et al. Neurological gait disorders in elderly people: clinical approach and classification. Lancet Neurol. 2007;6:63–74. https://doi.org/10.1016/S1474-4422(06)70678-0
Sudarsky L. Gait disorders in the elderly. NEJM. 1990;322:1441–1447. https://doi.org/10.1056/NEJM199005173222007

CASE 4

An older couple comes to your office seeking advice about exercise. The wife asks, "Doctor, would you please try to put some sense into my husband's head. He is 82 years old. All of a sudden, he wants to spend six hundred dollars to join a gym and start working out. Does that make sense?"

Questions

1. What more do you want to know about the patient's history, comorbidities, and social situation?

2. How would you go about performing an examination on this patient?

The patient tells you that he is healthy for his age. His only admission to the hospital was for an appendectomy. His only medications are amlodipine, hydrochlorothiazide, and atorvastatin. He is active in the house. He helps his wife with cleaning the house. He still likes to garden. He walks at an average pace in his neighborhood. There is one modest hill on his route. He can walk up a flight of stairs without difficulty. He would like to go to the gym and use the treadmill. He will set the speed at 3.5 miles per hour and raise the grade to an angle at which he feels that he is exercising but able to enjoy the work out without fatigue or exhaustion. He would like to use exercise stations in the gym for strength and tone.

His physical examination is normal for age.

3. What tests would you order?

4. What kind of exercise program would you prescribe?

5. The wife asks if anything can be done to reduce the amount of money that the husband is planning to spend.

6. The wife says this all sounds good, but will he develop arthritis?

Answers

1. Determine the patient's current level of activity. Is he sedentary or is he already exercising at home? Ask about the type of exercises that the patient might enjoy. Find out about household activities and the ability to walk, walk up stairs, or walk up hills that give some idea of the amount of activity, as measured by metabolic equivalent (MET) charts, that the patient is capable of. Obtain a full medical history, particularly asking about history of myocardial infarction, congestive heart failure, chronic obstructive pulmonary disease (COPD), peripheral vascular disease, stroke, joint disease, smoking, and diabetes. Perform a review of systems again looking for evidence of coronary artery disease, respiratory problems, peripheral vascular disease, or problems with the musculoskeletal system.

2. Perform a full physical examination. Document vital signs and body mass index. Examine the heart, lungs, and abdomen. Check pedal pulses. Examine the joints of the upper and lower extremities. Perform a neurologic examination looking for any deficit in cognition, cranial nerves, tone, reflexes, strength, sensation, balance, or coordination.

3. The patient describes activities that at about 4 METs. The American College of Cardiology recommends a stress test for:
   a. Men over the age 45 and women over the age of 55 who plan to exercise at 60% of VO2 max (maximum oxygen consumption).
   b. Anyone with symptoms of cardiac disease or known cardiac disease
   c. Anyone with symptoms of pulmonary disease
   d. Anyone with diabetes
   e. Anyone with two or more risk factors for cardiac disease.

   If the patient wants to walk in the neighborhood or the mall, he does not need a stress test. If he plans to walk on a treadmill with an uphill grade, a stress test would be prudent. A check of CBC, electrolytes, renal function, and hemoglobin A1C might be helpful.

4. A consensus panel from the American College of Sports Medicine and the American Heart Association recommends that patients of any age exercise 30 minutes every day if possible. The program should include aerobic exercises and exercises to maintain range of motion every day. Muscle strengthening should be performed 2 or 3 days per week. Exercise sessions should begin with stretching and warm-ups. Stretching should include static stretch to the muscles of the chest wall, hip flexors, hamstrings, and gastrocnemius muscles. Each muscle group should have a static stretch of 15 to 30 seconds that is repeated three times on each side of the body. Warm-up consists of beginning the cardiovascular activity at a slow pace. Moderate activity is defined as being at 60% to 80% of maximum heart rate or VO2 maximum. It may be easier for a patient to monitor their perceived level of exertion. On

a scale of 1 to 10, a rating of 5 or 6 corresponds with moderate activity and a rating of 7 or 8 with vigorous activity. Seniors may use the "talk test," which means that the participant is not too out of breath to comfortably talk. The aerobic session should end with a cooldown that is similar to the warm-up. Strengthening exercises should be done 2 to 3 nonconsecutive days per week. It is recommended that eight to 10 muscle groups be exercised. The weights should be light enough to allow 10 to 15 repetitions of each exercise with intensity of effort at about 5 to 6 on a 10-point scale. Strengthening exercises can reduce the decline in strength that occurs with aging. People tend to lose 15% of their strength per decade after age 50 and 30% per decade after age 70. Weight training prevents or reduces loss of bone mass and improves insulin sensitivity. Improvement in strength and balance reduces the risk of falling.

5. You ask the wife what type of insurance they have. Many Medicare Advantage plans include membership in a gym. Cost comparison shopping can find gyms with low monthly fees and no yearly contracts. If money is a real issue, seniors can do very well with walking in the neighborhood or malls and use of lightweights that can be purchased and used for many years.

6. You explain that contact sports and sports that involve frequent change of direction are associated with joint injury, but the program that you have described is not associated with increased development of osteoarthritis. In fact, moderate exercise has been shown to reduce the incidence of osteoarthritis of the hips and knees.

BIBLIOGRAPHY

Fiatarone MA, Marks EC, Ryan ND, et al. High Intensity training in nonagenarians. *JAMA*. 1990;263:3029–3034. https://doi.org/10.1001/jama.1990.03440220053029

Metsios GS, Stavropoulos-Kalinoglou A, Veldhuijzen van Zanten JJCS, et al. Rheumatoid arthritis, cardiovascular disease and physical exercise: a systematic review. *Rheumatology*. 2008;47:239–248. https://doi.org/10.1093/rheumatology/kem260

Neid RJ, Franklin B. Promoting and prescribing exercise for the elderly. *Am Fam Physician*. 2002;65:419–426.

Nelson ME, Rejeski WJ, Blair SN, et al. Physical activity and public health in older adults. Recommendations from the American College of Sports Medicine and the American Heart Association. *Circulation*. 2007;116:1094–1105. https://doi.org/10.1161/CIRCULATIONAHA.107.185650

8 Musculoskeletal Impairments

Michael Mallow

A 53-year-old woman presents to your outpatient office with a 6-month history of left shoulder pain and limited range of motion (ROM). She has never had this pain before, and it is interfering with her daily activities.

Questions

1. What more do you want to know about the patient's history, comorbidities, and social situation? Please tell me why you are asking for these specifics.

2. How would you go about performing a physical exam on this patient? Why are these maneuvers/exam components important?

She tells you that the pain is mainly in the anterior shoulder but can radiate all the way to her wrist. Pain is worsened with reaching, and she is very limited in her ability to reach overhead or behind her back. Cervical motion has no effect on her pain. The patient has a normal neurologic examination but significant restrictions in both active and passive ROM of the shoulder in all planes, especially with external rotation and abduction. She has pain with Hawkin's and Neer's maneuvers, but a negative empty can test. Her cervical ROM is full without reproduction of typical pain. Spurling's maneuver is negative.

3. What is the differential diagnosis for this patient? Tell me the most likely diagnosis and why.

4. What diagnostic test or tests would you order and why?

X-rays demonstrate mild degenerative changes in the acromioclavicular joint but an otherwise normal glenohumeral joint and no bony abnormality

5. Outline the treatment plan. Please tell me the initial treatment and next steps if that fails.

She works as a receptionist in a dental office. She asks whether this condition is work related and if she can make a workers' compensation claim. How should you respond?

6. How do you address her question?

The patient requests an MRI be ordered to make sure "nothing is torn."

7. Tell me in lay terms about . . . Or how would you respond to this request?

Answers

1. Key history elements include type of onset (insidious or traumatic), the main location of pain (anterior lateral shoulder, superior shoulder, scapular region), exacerbating factors (reaching overhead, behind), alleviating factors, any associated pain sleeping on the shoulder at night time (a common symptom of rotator cuff pathology), any symptoms worsened with cervical motion (to assess possible cervical source for pain), and underlying diabetes or thyroid disorders that can predispose the patient to adhesive capsulitis.

2. Essential examination elements include active and passive shoulder ROM, assessment of upper extremity strength, sensation, reflexes, presence of painful arc (60- to 120-degree shoulder abduction) that is seen in rotator cuff impingement, special shoulder tests (Hawkin's, Neer's, empty can), cervical spine ROM, palpation, and Spurling's maneuver.

3. Differential diagnosis includes rotator cuff impingement/tear, adhesive capsulitis, and glenohumeral osteoarthritis (OA).

4. X-ray of the shoulder should be obtained. Ultrasound of the shoulder may show tendinopathy of the rotator cuff. An MRI is not indicated at this time, given the lack of trauma and examination, as it would not change the clinical course at this point.

5. The patient likely has adhesive capsulitis. Patients with adhesive capsulitis generally present with restrictions in both active and passive ROM, as opposed to rotator cuff disease where active ROM is restricted but passive ROM is approximately normal. Glenohumeral OA can present with both passive and active ROM loss, but in this case, the absence of degenerative changes of the glenohumeral joint on x-rays make OA less likely. Discuss that the natural history resolves over 1 to 2 years. Most interventions have not been found to change the natural history. Treatment includes physical therapy focused on improving function, pain control, ROM, and scapular and rotator cuff strengthening. Oral analgesics for pain should be prescribed, usually nonsteroidals if no contraindications. Intra-articular injections of steroid or hydrodilation with large volumes of normal saline can be beneficial. Manipulation under anesthesia is reserved for refractory cases.

6. Get a thorough history of details of her job. A receptionist generally does not have excessive use of her shoulder to explain this. The patient's condition likely is covered by medical insurance but not workers' compensation. She can get unpaid time off from work for therapies or doctors' appointments under the Family Medical Leave Act.

7. Explain that her history and physical examination point to a diagnosis of adhesive capsulitis and that an MRI is not required at this time. Such tests are indicated when treatment fails and at this time, a tear of her rotator cuff, which is a common finding in people without shoulder pain, would not change the treatment plan.

BIBLIOGRAPHY

Andrews J. Frozen shoulder. In: Armstrong AD, Hubbard MC, eds. *Essentials of Musculoskeletal Care*. 3rd ed. American Academy of Orthopedic Surgeons; 2005:184–185.

Hsu JE, Anakwenze OA, Warrender WJ, et al. Current review of adhesive capsulitis. *J Shoulder Elbow Surg*. 2011;20(3):502–514. https://doi.org/10.1016/j.jse.2010.08.023

Rill BK, Fleckensetin CM, Levy MS, et al. Predictors of outcome after nonoperative and operative treatment of adhesive capsulitis. *Am J Sports Med*. 2011;39(3):567–574. https://doi.org/10.1177/0363546510385403

A 48-year-old, right-hand dominant electrician with a 5-month history of persistent pain in his right elbow presents to your office. The pain was of insidious onset with no precipitating injury or trauma. He is having difficulty performing his job duties, including gripping and using tools.

Questions

1. What more do you want to know about the patient's history, comorbidities, and social situation? Please tell me why you are asking for these specifics.

2. How would you go about performing a physical exam on this patient? Why are these maneuvers/exam components important?

He tells you the pain is mostly over the lateral aspect of his right elbow but does radiate along the lateral forearm. It had an insidious onset. He has no pain in the neck, arm, or beyond the wrist. He is an electrician. The patient has a normal neurologic examination. There is point tenderness over the lateral epicondyle, especially a few millimeters distal to the tip of the lateral epicondyle. Resisted wrist extension with the elbow extended and forearm pronated, resisted extension of the long finger, and maximal wrist flexion all increase pain at the lateral epicondyle.

3. What is the differential diagnosis for this patient? Tell me the most likely diagnosis and why.

4. What diagnostic test or tests would you order and why?

X-rays (anteroposterior [AP]/lateral of the elbow) were normal. A point-of-care limited diagnostic musculoskeletal ultrasound of the lateral elbow revealed hypoechoic swelling of the common extensor tendon (>4.2 mm) without an associated tear.

5. Outline the treatment plan. Please tell me the initial treatment and next steps if that fails.

He works as an electrician but is finding it difficult to perform his job duties.

6. What advice would you give him regarding activity modification and return to activity?

He appreciates your help but still seems unsure about the exact nature of the diagnosis and why the tear should not be surgically corrected.

7. Tell me the diagnosis in lay terms.

Answers

1. Key elements of the history include the location of the pain (diffuse pain over the lateral epicondyle and proximal forearm), type of onset (insidious versus traumatic; recent changes in training, technique, duties, or equipment used in sport or work), exacerbating factors (repetitive wrist extension, gripping), alleviating factors, severity of the pain, associated symptoms (absence of neck, upper thoracic, or shoulder pain; absence of sensory symptoms), and activity history (recent change in activities).

2. Essential examination elements include observation, active and passive elbow (flexion/extension, supination/pronation) and wrist (flexion/extension) ROM, resisted movements including wrist extension with the elbow extended and forearm pronated (Cozen test), grip test, resisted extension of the third metacarpophalangeal joint, palpation (lateral epicondyle, extensor muscles), and neurologic examination of the cervical spine (upper extremity strength, reflex, sensation testing).

3. The most likely diagnosis is lateral epicondylitis. The differential diagnosis includes referred pain from the cervical and upper thoracic spine, synovitis of the radiohumeral joint, radiohumeral bursitis, posterior interosseous nerve entrapment (radial tunnel syndrome), and osteochondritis dissecans.

4. Diagnostic tests are usually not needed but may be ordered to rule out other causes. These may include plain radiographs of the elbow (AP, lateral), diagnostic musculoskeletal ultrasound, and MRI imaging of the elbow.

5. Treatments include correcting predisposing factors, physical therapy (eccentric exercise program), therapeutic ultrasound, friction massage, counterforce bracing, wrist immobilization splints, and corticosteroid injection. There is a growing, though still controversial, body of evidence that platelet-rich plasma injections may help in refractory cases. Surgery is reserved for cases that fail conservative management.

6. It is important to correct predisposing factors. These may include equipment use such as modifying the type of screwdriver or other tools, changing grip size, and using proper mechanics. Return to work activities involving repetitive wrist extension and gripping should be gradual and take place over 3 to 6 weeks (varies depending on severity).

7. Describe lateral epicondylitis in lay terms as irritated tendon. Explain each treatment in eighth-grade language. Most people's symptoms go away in several weeks.

BIBLIOGRAPHY

Ihm J, Mautner K, Blazuk J, et al. Point/counterpoint. Platelet-rich plasma versus an eccentric exercise program for recalcitrant lateral elbow tendinopathy. *PM R.* 2015;7(6):654–661. https://doi.org/10.1016/j.pmrj.2015.05.001

Scott A, Bell S, Vicenzino B. Elbow and arm pain. In: Brukner P, Khan K, eds. *Brukner & Khan's Clinical Sports Medicine.* 4th ed. McGraw-Hill Education; 2012:390–401.

Woodley BL, Newsham-West RJ, Baxter GD. Chronic tendinopathy: effectiveness of eccentric exercise. *Br J Sports Med.* 2007;41(4):188–198; discussion 199. https://doi.org/10.1136/bjsm.2006.029769

Mr. James is a 67-year-old gentleman who presents with chronic bilateral knee pain. The pain started 5 years ago and is progressive. Currently, the pain is worse with movement and improved with rest. He does admit the right knee has been swollen off and on during the last 3 months.

Questions

1. What more do you want to know about the patient's history, comorbidities, and social situation? Please tell me why you are asking for these specifics.

2. How would you go about performing a physical exam on this patient? Why are these maneuvers/exam components important?

There is a 2+ effusion to the right knee and a trace effusion on the left. McMurray's test is positive bilaterally. Strength is 5/5. Some redness surrounds the right knee.

3. What is the differential diagnosis for this patient? Tell me the most likely diagnosis and why.

4. What diagnostic test or tests would you order and why?

X-rays show moderate OA and right knee effusion.

5. Outline the treatment plan. Please tell me the initial treatment and next steps if that fails.

Mr. James returns after 2 weeks and complains that pain and decreased ROM limit his participation in therapy (or home exercise). He asks if an MRI is reasonable or if there is anything else you can do for the pain.

6. How do you address his question?

Mr. James returns in 6 weeks as scheduled. He is feeling 60% better. A physician friend of his ordered an MRI of his right knee, and he provides you with the study. The images and report indicate a right medial meniscal tear. He asks for the name of an orthopedic surgeon for potential knee arthroscopy.

7. How would you respond?

Answers

1. Did the patient have any trauma, fever, chills, or locking or catching of the knee on flexion and extension? This is critical to build a differential diagnosis of the injury and triage diagnostic plans.

2. Examinations should include strength, ROM, inspection, palpation, and special tests for meniscal pathology.

3. The most likely situation is that he is suffering from knee OA. An acute injury such as a fracture, ligament, or meniscus is unlikely given the time course.

4. An x-ray of the knee is reasonable to assess the severity of knee OA. An MRI would not be indicated in this case given no mechanical symptoms (locking or catching) and no concern for ligamentous injury that would require surgical consideration.

5. A course of physical therapy or home exercise would be reasonable with the provision of a nonsteroidal anti-inflammatory drug (NSAID) or Tylenol. Opiate pain medications would be less than ideal at this point. Draining the right knee with a corticosteroid injection in the right knee and/or the left knee is reasonable; however, x-rays should be obtained first.

6. As earlier, an MRI would not be indicated in this case given no mechanical symptoms (locking or catching) and no concern for ligamentous injury that would require surgical consideration.

7. It should be explained to Mr. James that there is no evidence that arthroscopic surgery is helpful for an atraumatic meniscal tear. There is a very high rate of asymptomatic tears, and the tear apparent on MRI may not be causing his pain. After this explanation, the name of a surgeon or orthopedic practice should, of course, be provided at the patient's request for a second opinion.

BIBLIOGRAPHY

Bhattacharyya T, Gale D, Dewire P, et al. The clinical importance of meniscal tears demonstrated by magnetic resonance imaging in osteoarthritis of the knee. *J Bone Joint Surg Am.* 2003;85-A:4–9. https://doi.org/10.2106/00004623-200301000-00002

Hepper CT, Halvorson JJ, Duncan ST, et al. The efficacy and duration of injection for knee osteoarthritis. *Sport Med.* 2009;17(10):638–646. https://doi.org/10.5435/00124635-200910000-00006

Krych AJ, Johnson NR, Mohan R, et al. Partial meniscectomy provides no benefit for symptomatic degenerative medial meniscus posterior root tears. *Knee Surg Sports Traumatol Arthrosc.* February 9, 2017. https://doi.org/10.1007/s00167-017-4454-5

Uthman I, Raynauld J-P, Haraoui B. Intra-articular therapy in osteoarthritis. *Postgrad Med J.* 2003;79(934):449–453. https://doi.org/10.1136/pmj.79.934.449

CASE 4

A 72-year-old man who is an avid golfer comes to your office with a chief complaint of right shoulder pain and weakness for 4 weeks.

Questions

1. What more do you want to know about the patient's history, comorbidities, and social situation? Please tell me why you are asking for these specifics.

2. How would you go about performing a physical exam on this patient? Why are these maneuvers/exam components important?

There was no acute trauma. The pain came on gradually and is located in the anterior aspect of the right shoulder. No radiation of pain into the right hand is described. Pain is worse with overhead activities. He lacks full active ROM on the right in abduction. Strength in external rotation on the right is 2+/5. Impingement signs are positive, as is the drop arm test. There is moderate scapular dyskinesis.

3. What is the differential diagnosis for this patient? Tell me the most likely diagnosis and why.

4. What diagnostic test or tests would you order and why?

The patient returns in 1 week and is still complaining of pain. His primary physician ordered an MRI at his request, and it shows a partial tear of the right supraspinatus.

5. Outline the treatment plan. Please tell me the initial treatment and next steps if that fails.

He would very much like to return to golf as soon as possible.

6. What are return-to-play guidelines for the patient to resume his golf game?

He continues to have trouble understanding why the tear should not be fixed surgically.

7. Explain in lay terms the thinking in this situation.

Answers

1. History should include recent trauma, prior injury, prior and current function, character and location of pain, exacerbating and remitting factors, and radiation of pain.

2. Examination should include strength testing, sensory examination, reflexes, shoulder and neck active and passive ROM, and assessment of scapular motion.

3. Differential diagnosis includes rotator cuff tear, impingement syndrome, acromioclavicular joint arthritis, and glenohumeral joint arthritis.

4. The patient should be referred for physical therapy including rotator cuff strengthening. He should also be offered treatment for his pain and discomfort. Next steps may include ultrasound or MRI, but that would be unlikely to change management at this time given that this is an atraumatic tear in a patient who should start a conservative course of care prior to consideration of operative repair.

5. Management does not change. There is no evidence to support operative management of atraumatic rotator cuff tears.

6. Prior to a gradual return to sport, he should exhibit improved strength and mobility. A gradual, sport-specific, return should then be discussed.

7. Use terms appropriate to the situation (e.g., lay language) to explain that our understanding of his injury, based on the study of patients with his condition, shows that rotator cuff tearing is relatively common and responds well to conservative care.

BIBLIOGRAPHY

Kibler WB, Murrell AC. Shoulder pain. In Brukner P, Khan K, eds. *Brukner & Khan's Clinical Sports Medicine.* 4th ed. McGraw-Hill; 2012:242–289.

Tashjian RZ. Epidemiology, natural history, and indications for treatment of rotator cuff tears. *Clin Sports Med.* 2012;31(4):589–604. https://doi.org/10.1016/j.csm.2012.07.001

Tempelhof S, Rupp S, Seil R. Age-related prevalence of rotator cuff tears in asymptomatic shoulders. *J Shoulder Elbow Surg.* 1999;8(4):296–299. https://doi.org/10.1016/S1058-2746(99)90148-9

CASE 5

A 22-year-old male presents to your clinic with an acute right ankle injury. When playing tennis the day before, he pushed off and felt immediate sharp right posterior ankle pain. There was an audible pop at the onset of pain.

Questions

1. What more do you want to know about the patient's history, comorbidities, and social situation? Please tell me why you are asking for these specifics.

2. How would you go about performing a physical exam on this patient? Why are these maneuvers/exam components important?

He complains of sharp ankle pain and has limited ability to ambulate in the office. His ankle is in plantar flexion as he sits on the examination table. Thompson's test is positive. There is tenderness on gentle palpation of the Achilles tendon.

3. What is the differential diagnosis for this patient? Tell me the most likely diagnosis and why.

4. What diagnostic test or tests would you order and why?

X-ray obtained in the office is normal. Bedside ultrasound examination shows a nearly complete tear of the right Achilles tendon.

5. Outline the treatment plan. Please tell me the initial treatment and next steps if that fails.

The patient tells you that he has limited insurance coverage and feels he will be unable to make an appointment with orthopedics or afford surgery.

6. How do you proceed?

He thanks you for the offer of support but is still concerned about costs. He has learned that it is possible to treat this injury nonoperatively and asks that you prescribe that treatment.

7. How do you respond?

Answers

1. It is important to inquire about associate injuries such as a fall or possible ankle fracture. A functional history is also important with respect to short-term management.

2. Thompson's test allows the examiner to assess for an Achilles tendon injury. In a complete tear, compression/squeeze of the calf will not case ankle plantar flexion.

3. Given the history and examination, this represents a likely complete Achilles tendon tear. Other possibilities include ankle fracture, Achilles tendinopathy, gastrocnemius strain, and peroneal tendon tear.

4. An x-ray of the ankle is reasonable to rule out associate osseous injury. The Achilles tendon should be imaged either by musculoskeletal ultrasound or MRI, depending on local resources.

5. Initial treatment should include fracture boot immobilization with a heel lift and the provision of crutches. Orthopedic consultation should be arranged so that the patient can discuss operative versus nonoperative care.

6. Providing empathy in this situation is important. The patient should have a surgical consultation, and the provider should help the patient navigate the local healthcare system. If the patient does have insurance, his company can be contacted to provide orthopedic consultation options. Options include a social work consultation if available, personal discussion with a local orthopedist, or discussion with clinic or hospital administration to find the options.

7. Given the patient's age and injury (complete tear), a conversation with a surgeon is important so that he can appropriately understand the options in front of him, including the operative recovery process. His wishes should, of course, be acknowledged; however, the examiner should make it clear that the recommendation is for orthopedic consultation and that help will be provided to make that happen.

BIBLIOGRAPHY

Okewunmi J, Guzman J, Vulcano E. Achilles tendinosis injuries-tendinosis to rupture (getting the athlete back to play). *Clin Sports Med.* 2020;39(4). https://doi.org/10.1016/j.csm.2020.05.001

Patel KA, O'Malley MJ. Management of Achilles tendon injuries in the elite athlete. *Orthop Clin North Am.* 2020;51(4):533–539, 877–891. https://doi.org/10.1016/j.ocl.2020.06.009

CASE 6

A new first-time mother presents to your outpatient office with right wrist pain for the last 3 weeks. There has been no trauma, but she notes that she is bottle-feeding her child. She feels most of the pain on the radial aspect of her wrist.

Questions

1. What more do you want to know about the patient's history, comorbidities, and social situation? Please tell me why you are asking for these specifics.

2. How would you go about performing a physical exam on this patient? Why are these maneuvers/exam components important?

She tried an over-the counter (OTC) splint for the last 2 weeks without improvement and has used ice and NSAIDs (she is not nursing). She describes a limitation of activities at home, including struggling to change the baby's diaper. She has tenderness to palpation of the right wrist, near the radial styloid. Slight swelling is noted. Finkelstein's test is positive.

3. What is the differential diagnosis for this patient? Tell me the most likely diagnosis and why.

4. What diagnostic test or tests would you order and why?

De Quervain's tenosynovitis is primarily a clinical diagnosis, and no additional testing is required.

5. Outline the treatment plan. Please tell me the initial treatment and next steps if that fails.

During most of the visit, you notice that the patient appears fatigued and makes limited eye contact. She opens up a bit and admits that she has felt "down" lately since the birth of her child but has a lot of support from her family.

6. How would you respond to this statement?

She states that she had felt depressed before and was in therapy, but "it wasn't like this." She denies suicidal ideation (SI) or homicidal ideation (HI) but admits to sleeping very poorly (2–3 hours a day) and lacking interest in activities she normally enjoys. She becomes tearful during this discussion.

7. How do you proceed?

Answers

1. A functional history should be obtained with respect to possible contributing activities and current limitations, as this will drive management decisions. The provider should obtain a detailed assessment of other treatments that have been employed. It is important to understand what type of brace she attempted to use.

2. Inspection and gentle palpation of the wrist should be done, as well as reproduction of pain with wrist active and passive ROM. Finkelstein's is commonly done to assess for de Quervain's tenosynovitis. It is positive when pain is reproduced with the wrist in ulnar deviation while the thumb is held in the patient's closed hand.

3. De Quervain's tenosynovitis is the most likely diagnosis given the location of pain and examination. Other possibilities include tendinopathy, occult trauma, and degenerative conditions.

4. De Quervain's tenosynovitis is a clinical diagnosis. It is not unreasonable to obtain an x-ray of the hand/wrist, but it is not required. MRI imaging would be very unlikely to change the treatment plan at this point, prior to the start of some conservative care, and should not be ordered.

5. The treatment of de Quervain's tenosynovitis is somewhat varied, with some recommending splinting and rest prior to the initiation of a corticosteroid injection while others point to evidence supporting early use of injection therapy. In this setting, where some conservative treatment has been attempted by the patient, and given that her pain is significant, an injection is reasonable.

6. The patient's current mental health state should be fully assessed.

7. Postpartum depression is a serious issue and should be treated as such. Empathy is important, but also it is important to have a specific conversation about resources. It should be determined what support she has for mental health and appropriate assistance be provided to accessing those services. Simply giving her a phone number is not sufficient.

BIBLIOGRAPHY

Awan WA, Babur MN, Masood T. Effectiveness of therapeutic ultrasound with or without thumb spica splint in the management of De Quervain's disease. *J Back Musculoskelet Rehabil.* 2017;30(4):691–697. https://doi.org/10.3233/BMR-160591

Blood TD, Morrell NT, Weiss APC. Tenosynovitis of the hand and wrist: a critical analysis review. *JBJS Review.* 2016;4(3). https://doi.org/10.2106/JBJS.RVW.O.00061

Roh YH, Hong SW, Gong HS, et al. Ultrasound-guided versus blind corticosteroid injections for De Quervain tendinopathy: a prospective randomized trial. *J Hand Surg Eur Vol.* 2018;43(8):820–824. https://doi.org/10.1177/1753193418790535

9 Neuromuscular Impairments and Electrodiagnosis

Tae Hwan Chung

A 55-year-old man comes to a neuromuscular clinic complaining of numbness and burning sensation in both feet. The symptom started about 2 years ago, and he has no other known past medical history.

Questions

1. What questions would you ask before planning for further diagnostic workup?

2. What physical exam findings are important?

You learn that his symptoms started gradually about 2 years ago in the bottom of his feet, and slowly progressed to the mid-shin level. It started with severe burning, followed by numbness, and he also feels some weakness in the ankles. The symptoms progressed symmetrically. More recently, he started having some urinary retention and severe constipation. He became a vegan at age 50 to improve his health. He is having trouble in his work as a real estate agent due to limited walking tolerance. His wife says he has become forgetful and clumsy in the past few months. He has no family history of neurologic disease. His exam shows normal strength, except for 4/5 in the dorsiflexion and plantarflexion of both ankles. Sensory deficits are in a length-dependent pattern for all sensory modalities. Proprioception is poor in both great toes. Vibration sense is absent below the knees. Deep tendon reflexes (DTRs) are absent in both ankles, but 3+ in the knees with positive cross-adductor responses bilaterally. He was able to recall one object out of three in a short-term memory test, but his long-term memory is intact.

3. What is in the differential?

4. What diagnostic tests are indicated?

His nerve conduction study (NCS) shows absent sural sensory response, low compound motor action potential (CMAP) amplitudes of bilateral peroneal at extensor digiti brevis (EDB), and bilateral tibial nerves, whereas the motor response of bilateral peroneal at tibialis anterior are normal. Electromyography (EMG) shows mild spontaneous activities and several large units with a neurogenic recruitment pattern in the tibialis anterior and gastrocnemius muscles, but other muscles are normal. His labs show borderline low-serum vitamin B12 level but very high-serum methylmalonic acid (MMA) and high-serum homocysteine levels. MRI of the brain and spinal cord is normal.

5. What is the diagnosis, and what treatment would you recommend?

6. If he were a vegan for religious reasons, how might you approach the conversation differently?

At the end of the visit, he reveals that he has been a strict vegan for several years since his brother died of a massive stroke, and he wants to have your opinions on his diet.

7. Explain to him how his diet affects this disorder?

Answers

1. Ask about weakness, numbness, and pain. Ask about exposure to toxins, chemotherapy, and other medications. A thorough review of systems to exclude systemic disease is important. Ask about family history of neurologic disease (e.g., Charcot-Marie-Tooth).

2. Important physical exam findings include DTRs; manual muscle testing; sensory exam with light touch, pinprick, and vibration/position; and brief memory test.

3. Differential diagnosis includes polyneuropathy, myelopathy, subacute combined degeneration, entrapment neuropathy, neuroma, complex regional pain syndrome (CRPS), and multilevel lumbosacral radiculopathy.

4. Tests indicated include EMG/NCS; complete blood count (CBC); vitamin B1, B6, and B12 levels; hemoglobin A1c (HbA1c; or blood sugar level); MRI of spine; and MRI of brain.

5. EMG/NCS shows a length-dependent sensorimotor polyneuropathy; he has subacute combined degeneration from vitamin B12 deficiency, given high MMA and homocysteine level (when serum vitamin B12 is borderline low, MMA and homocysteine levels are more sensitive, especially when serum level of vitamin B12 is borderline low). Treatment includes intramuscular vitamin B12 injection for 1 month, followed by oral vitamin B12 supplement; physical therapy (PT) for strengthening and balance training; and orthotic evaluation if patient has neurological gait dysfunction.

6. If his veganism was due to religious or moral considerations, you should be nonjudgmental about his diet and can advise him that supplementation with B12 is necessary.

7. He has subacute combined degeneration from B12 deficiency. His peripheral neuropathy from vitamin B12 is likely due to his veganism, given the timeline. The advice to this patient should include (a) risks of extreme diet habits; (b) referral to nutritionist; (c) importance of exercise, in addition to diet, for cardiovascular health; (d) communicating with his primary physician regarding his cardiovascular risks and the family history; and (e) dietary recommendations for B12-rich foods.

BIBLIOGRAPHY

Amato AA, Dumitru D. Approach to peripheral neuropathy. In: Dumitru D, ed. *Electrodiagnostic Medicine*. 2nd ed. Hanley & Belfus; 2002:chap 21.

Amato AA, Russell JA. Neuropathies associated with systemic disorder. In: Amato AA, Russell JA, eds. *Neuromuscular Disorder*. McGraw-Hill; 2008:chap 14.

Dombovy ML. Rehabilitation management of neuropathies. In: Dyck PJ, Thomas PK, eds. *Peripheral Neuropathy*. 4th ed. Elsevier; 2005:2621–2636. https://doi.org/10.1016/B978-0-7216-9491-7.50120-4

CASE 2

A 62-year-old female with progressive muscle weakness is referred to your physical medicine and rehabilitation (PM&R) clinic. She started having muscle weakness after spine surgery performed about 3 years ago, and now she uses a wheelchair for mobility. She recently developed difficulty swallowing and has a soft voice.

Questions

1. What questions would you ask before planning for further diagnostic workup?

2. What are the important physical findings?

She says that she developed right foot drop about 3 years ago, but there was no sensory deficits. She always had very mild back pain, and her neurosurgeon decided to perform spine surgery. However, after the surgery, the weakness worsened and progressed to the right knee, left ankle, and the right hip over the next 1 to 2 years. About a year ago, she developed right wrist drop and some weakness in the left elbow. There has been no sensory deficits or changes in the back pain. On exam she has brisk reflexes, including a jaw jerk. She has atrophy of both upper and lower limbs and fasciculation of her tongue and quadriceps.

3. Please list the differential diagnosis.

4. What other diagnostic workups would you recommend, and what is the rationale?

You decided to do an electrodiagnostic study. The NCS shows normal sensory studies in both lower and upper extremities. However, CMAPs of the peroneal, tibial, and right radial motor nerves are all reduced with relatively preserved conduction velocity in an asymmetric pattern. EMG shows 3 to 4+ spontaneous activities and very large units with the neurogenic recruitment pattern in all the muscles from the bulbar, cervical, thoracic, and lumbosacral regions. Fasciculation potentials are frequently seen in multiple muscles. All the labs and imaging studies came back negative.

5. What is the presumed diagnosis? What is your approach to the patient for prognostication and what is your treatment plan for her?

At the follow-up visit, she says she recently saw an alternative medicine doctor who says her amyotrophic lateral sclerosis (ALS) is related to a subclinical Lyme infection, although she never had any positive Lyme test. She is considering receiving intravenous (IV) doxycycline for 6 months as recommended by the doctor.

6. What advice would you give to her?

7. Explain the disease and prognosis to her in lay terms.

Answers

1. Questions should involve the time course/progression of symptoms; distribution of sensory symptoms, if any; distribution of motor deficits; how the symptoms limit her daily functions; possible complications from the spine surgery; and progression of back pain. How is this impacting her participation in daily activities?

2. The important physical findings are DTRs, upper motor neuron signs (at least two of the following should be done: cross-adduction, Babinski, Hoffman's, jaw jerk), manual muscle testing, sensory exam, inspection of tongue for fasciculation and/or atrophy, and inspection for fasciculation and/or atrophy in limb and trunk muscles.

3. Differential diagnosis includes ALS, multilevel radiculopathy, vasculitic neuropathy, and inclusion body myositis.

4. Workup: CBC and metabolic panel, toxicity screening (including heavy metal), creatine phosphokinase (CPK) (and/or aldolase), cerebrospinal fluid (CSF) analysis, MRI of spine and MRI of brain, and electrodiagnostic studies.

5. The patient meets the El Escorial criteria for the diagnosis of ALS. Treatment plans should include the following: palliative care; riluzole; aggressive pulmonary rehabilitation (should mention continuous positive airway pressure [CPAP] and/or bilevel positive airway pressure [BiPAP] ± CoughAssist); speech evaluation for dysphagia and communication; wheelchair evaluation; PT evaluation for mobility; and occupational therapy (OT) evaluation for activities of daily living (ADLs) and adaptive devices.

6. While the association between chronic Lyme and ALS may be controversial, this patient never had a Lyme infection, given the negative Lyme tests. It should be clearly mentioned that the potential risks of IV doxycycline treatment in the absence of Lyme infection will outweigh any potential benefits of the treatment. The consultation should include the following: scientific rationale for alternative treatments; potential risks of alternative treatments; ethical and legal issues involving alternative treatments; and financial issues with alternative care. You should sensitively counsel the patient that many people may offer unproven treatments for her disease and that she should carefully weigh the evidence for their efficacy and the risks versus benefits.

7. It is important to clearly inform the patient in a sensitive way that ALS is a fatal disease with a median life span of fewer than 5 years. You might start by asking the patient how much she wants to know about the prognosis now. You can emphasize that we can only give average life spans, and that there are some people who are long-term survivors (e.g., Stephen Hawking). You should also initiate a conversation about advance directives. Would she want enteral feedings or home mechanical ventilation?

BIBLIOGRAPHY

Amato AA, Russell JA. Amyotrophic lateral sclerosis. In: Amato AA, Russell JA, eds. *Neuromuscular Disorder.* McGraw-Hill; 2008:chap 4.

de Carvalho M, Dengler R, Eisen A, et al. Electrodiagnostic criteria for diagnosis of ALS. *Clin Neurophys.* 2008;119:497–503. https://doi.org/10.1016/j.clinph.2007.09.143

Howard RS. Respiratory failure because of neuromuscular disease. *Curr Opin Neurol.* October 2016;29(5):592–601. https://doi.org/10.1097/WCO.0000000000000363

Kiernan MC, Vucic S. Amyotrophic lateral sclerosis. *Lancet.* March 12, 2011;377(9769):942–955. https://doi.org/10.1016/S0140-6736(10)61156-7

A 43-year-old female with progressive muscle weakness in her shoulders and hips is referred to your PM&R clinic. She developed muscle weakness about 3 months ago. She also noticed some skin lesions but denies any pain.

Questions

1. What questions would you ask before planning for further diagnostic workup?

2. What are the important physical findings?

She says that she realized one day that she could not comb her hair or stand up from a toilet by herself. She developed the weakness over 3 to 5 days but did not have any pain. A few days later, she developed rashes and severe itchiness in the face and knuckles. She has proximal muscle weakness. Reflexes are normal and she has no upper motor neuron signs.

3. What is the differential diagnosis?

4. What diagnostic tests would you order?

A sensory conduction study is normal, but EMG shows small units with early recruitment patterns in proximal muscles (Figure 9.1). A muscle biopsy shows extensive inflammation in the perimysium and endomysium, with perifascicular atrophy (Figure 9.2).

5. What is the diagnosis? What is the next step of workup and treatment? What are potential complications of treatment?

At the follow-up visit, you notice that her weakness has declined again. She admits that she has been skipping her medications

6. What would you advise her?

7. Explain her diagnosis and treatment to her in lay terms.

Answers

1. Questions involve the time course/progression of symptoms; distribution of sensory symptoms, if any; distribution of muscle weakness; how the symptoms limit her daily functions; any skin lesions; and any joint pain.

2. Physical findings include DTRs, manual muscle testing, and sensory exam inspection of skin lesions.

3. Differential diagnosis includes dermatomyositis, polymyositis, inclusion body myositis, toxic myopathy, and transverse myelitis.

4. Workup includes EMG/NCS; myositis-specific antibodies; CPK (and/or aldolase); MRI of muscle; MRI of spine, muscle biopsy.

5. Initial treatment is with high-dose steroids and an immune modulator such as mycophenylate. Exercise is helpful in regaining muscle strength. However, patients often develop steroid myopathy after several months of treatment. On the other hand, if steroids are tapered too rapidly, patients may develop Addison's syndrome (hypoaldosteronism). Depression is also common.

6. Patient education about the importance of immune medications and their potential benefits/risks should be the first step. Ask if her insurance covers the medicine and how high the co-pay is. Is this the issue? If appropriate, referral to social services can be considered. Some pharmaceutical companies offer discounts for patients with financial difficulties.

7. You need to use eighth grade-level language and elicit whether she understands what you have explained. Talk about the body's immune system attacking her muscle cells and how medication stops this process.

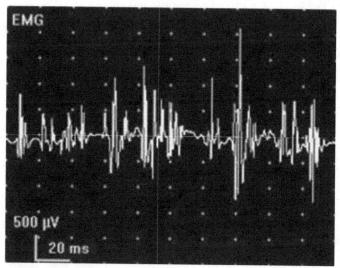

EMG, electromyogram.

Figure 9.1 EMG small-amplitude polyphasic motor unit.

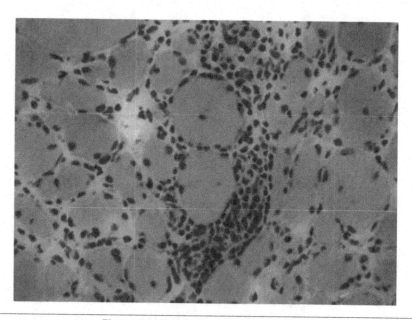

Figure 9.2 Muscle biopsy dermatomyositis.

Figure 9.5. ...

A right-handed, 33-year-old male is referred to your EMG clinic for evaluation of numbness and tingling in the right hand. He also has occasional neck pain. He is a software engineer who works on a computer all day long.

Questions

1. What questions would you ask before planning for further diagnostic workup?

2. What are the important physical exam findings and why? What is the most important diagnostic test to order?

He says the pain started about 1 year ago but worsened about 6 months ago. He drops things at work. He sometimes wakes up at night due to pain. He is having trouble typing. He has a positive Tinel's and Phalen's test, but negative Spurling's and Hoffman's tests.

3. What is the differential diagnosis? What is the most likely diagnosis?

4. How would you approach the electrodiagnostic studies?

In the electrodiagnostic study, the right median sensory conduction study shows reduction of the conduction velocity across the wrist, while the left side is normal. CMAP of the right median nerve shows distal latency of 6.0 ms (normal <4.2 ms), and amplitudes are more than 50% reduced in the right side compared to the left side (5 mV vs. 12 mV). Sensory and motor conduction studies of ulnar and radial nerves are all normal bilaterally. EMG of the abductor digiti minimi and flexor digitorum longus showed no abnormalities.

5. What are the treatment options for this patient?

6. What are appropriate work restrictions or accommodations for this patient?

Suppose during the needle EMG of the abductor pollicis brevis muscle, the patient suddenly becomes very anxious due to pain, screaming to stop the EMG study.

7. How would you communicate with the patient about the importance of concluding the test?

Answers

1. Questions include time course/progression of symptoms; distribution of sensory symptoms, if any; distribution of motor deficits; how the symptoms limit his daily functions; and the nature of neck pain (radiation, distribution, and frequency).

2. The exam should be focused on common entrapment neuropathy (carpal tunnel and/or cubital tunnel syndrome) and cervical radiculopathy, especially at the C8T1 level. Tests should address DTRs; manual muscle testing of median versus ulnar versus radial nerve innervated muscles; sensory exam of median versus ulnar versus radial nerve distribution; inspection of muscle atrophy in the median or ulnar innervated muscles; Tinel's signs at the wrist or elbow. Phalen's sign should also be checked, as it is more sensitive than the Tinel's sign. Any physical exam for cervical radiculopathy should include range of motion, Spurling's signs, and Hoffman's signs.

3. Differential diagnosis includes carpal tunnel syndrome (most likely) and other median nerve entrapments such as space-occupying lesions, cervical radiculopathy, thoracic outlet syndrome, and peripheral neuropathy.

4. NCS should include either a comparison of median nerve sensory latencies to the radial nerve at the thumb or alternatively wrist to mid palmar stimulation. Motor conduction can help with prognostication. Needle electromyography should at a minimum include at least one distal median-innervated muscle (abductor pollicus brevis), one ulnar-mediated muscle (such as first dorsal interosseous or abductor digiti minimi), and one median-innervated muscle proximal to carpal tunnel (such as pronator teres). Ideally, a sampling of C5-T1 muscles and paraspinals can be done to exclude cervical radiculopathy.

5. Splinting is the most reasonable first step. However, given that he has at least moderate severity carpal tunnel syndrome (with motor involvement), surgical consultation for carpal tunnel release should be considered. Other interventions might include ergonomic modification, occupational hand therapy, corticosteroid injection, median nerve gliding exercise, and pain medications (including nonsteroidal anti-inflammatory drugs [NSAIDs]).

6. Explore whether using voice-activated typing would work for him. Adjustments can be made to his keyboard and mouse to make them more ergonomic. He should take frequent rest breaks from typing.

7. If the patient has a decision-making capacity, the examiner should respect his wishes and stop the procedure. However, the disadvantage of stopping the procedure should be explained to the patient, and if necessary, the study should be reattempted. If the patient still refuses the procedure, alternative options should be provided. To minimize the discomfort, the following can be

considered: planning to do needling of the most painful muscles at the end, distraction technique by talking to the patient during the procedure, providing calm environment, and clear prior explanation of the procedure.

BIBLIOGRAPHY

Amato AA, Russell JA. Cervical and thoracic radiculopathies, brachial plexopathies, and mononeuropathies of the arm. In: Amato AA, Russell JA, eds. *Neuromuscular Disorder*. McGraw-Hill; 2008:chap 21.

American Association of Electrodiagnostic Medicine, American Academy of Neurology, and American Academy of Physical Medicine and Rehabilitation. Practice parameter for electrodiagnostic studies in carpal tunnel syndrome: summary statement. *Muscle Nerve*. 2009;25:918–922. https://doi.org/10.1002/mus.10185

Huisstede BM, Hoogvliet P, Randsdorp MS, et al. Carpal tunnel syndrome. Part I: effectiveness of nonsurgical treatments: a systemic review. *Arch Phys Med Rehab*. 2010;91(7):981–1004. https://doi.org/10.1016/j.apmr.2010.03.022

Huisstede BM, Randsdorp MS, Coert JH, et al. Carpal tunnel syndrome. Part II: effectiveness of surgical treatments: a systemic review. *Arch Phys Med Rehab*. 2010;91(7):1005–1024. https://doi.org/10.1016/j.apmr.2010.03.023

CASE 5

A 57-year-old male presents with generalized weakness and droopy eyes. He developed the symptoms about 3 months ago. He denies any numbness or tingling sensation.

Questions

1. What questions would you ask before planning for further diagnostic workup?

2. What are the important physical findings and diagnostic workup? Provide a rationale for each workup as well.

He says that he first developed droopiness in his eyes, especially in the evening. About 3 months ago, he developed fatigue that worsens toward the evening. In the morning, he can do most ADLs without difficulty, but throughout the day, he develops difficulty with lifting his arms above his head and his legs feel very heavy. By evening, his eyes become droopy to the point where he cannot see. He also noticed that he has double vision in the evening. Physical exam showed proximal muscle weakness with intact sensory function and normal, symmetric DTRs. Ice test improved ptosis.

3. What is the differential diagnosis?

4. What are the next steps of workup?

When he tried edrophonium for a few days, he felt improved energy overall and resolution of ptosis. An NCS is normal. EMG is also normal. However, a repetitive stimulation test shows decremental response but absence of postexercise facilitation. Lab also showed high-titer acetylcholine receptor antibody.

5. What is the diagnosis? Describe the treatment plan, including the role of exercise.

He returns to clinic after beginning treatments and is feeling better. He wants to join a health club to exercise more and lose weight. He brings a medical release form from the gym.

6. How would you handle this situation?

7. Explain his diagnosis and treatment to him in lay terms.

Answers

1. Questions involve the time course/progression of symptoms; distribution of muscle weakness; presence of visual or oculomotor symptoms; how the symptoms limit her daily functions; any skin lesions; and any joint pain.

2. Physical findings include DTRs, manual muscle testing, oculomotor, and sensory exam. Ice test can be considered; an ice pack is applied to the affected eyelid for 2 to 5 minutes to see if it improves ptosis by >2 mm or more. Also check for neck mass for thymoma. Workup includes EMG/NCS with repetitive simulation test. Labs should include auto-antibody against acetylcholine receptor and MuSK (muscle-specific tyrosine kinase). Finally, a therapeutic and diagnostic trial of edrophonium can be considered.

3. The differential diagnosis would include myasthenia gravis (most likely), Eaton–Lambert syndrome, and the Miller–Fisher variant of Guillain-Barré. One would worry about a paraneoplastic syndrome with his cough and weight loss.

4. Electrodiagnostic studies with repetitive stimulation and/or single-fiber EMG are essential in the diagnosis of myasthenia gravis. They can also help exclude amyotrophic lateral sclerosis (ALS) or Guillian-Barré Syndrome (GBS). One should check for acetylcholine antibodies. A paraneoplastic workup with PET-CT may be warranted. At the very least, a CT chest should look for thymoma, which is associated with MG. An edrophonium trial is also helpful in confirming the diagnosis.

5. Myasthenia gravis is the diagnosis. Treatment includes prednisone (steroid) followed by a secondary agent (i.e., intravenous immunoglobulin [IVIG], Imuran, methotrexate, or rituximab). If the repetitive stimulation and labs were normal, a single-fiber EMG should be considered when clinical symptoms are still suggestive of a neuromuscular junction disorder. In addition, a CT scan should be done to evaluate for a thymoma. If thymoma is present, thymectomy is generally recommended. The role of therapeutic exercise is unclear. Intense exercise is contraindicated as it can cause exacerbation.

6. You should either refuse to sign the form or indicate strict precautions for it. Offer the patient the alternative of beginning his exercise program under the supervision of a physical therapist, where the safety of the program can be assessed by a professional.

7. You need to use eighth grade-level language and elicit whether he understands what you have explained. Talk about the body's immune system attacking a structure called the neuromuscular junction, where nerve and muscle communicate with each other, and how medication stops this process.

BIBLIOGRAPHY

Amato AA, Russell JA. Disorders of neuromuscular transmission. In: Amato AA, Russell JA, eds. *Neuromuscular Disorder*. McGraw-Hill; 2008:chap 23.

Gilhus NE. Myasthenia gravis. *N Engl J Med*. December 29, 2016;375(26):2570–2581. https://doi.org/10.1056/NEJMra1602678. PMID: 28029925.

A 28-year-old male comes to your clinic complaining of weakness in the right shoulder in addition to mild numbness in the right shoulder area that started about 3 months ago.

Questions

1. What questions would you ask before planning for further diagnostic workup?

2. What are the important physical findings?

He says that he developed severe pain in the right shoulder 1 week ago. He had no trauma, and symptoms started suddenly in the middle of the day. He began to notice weakness about 3 days ago. He has difficulty lifting his right arm. He has no skin lesions. The sensory deficit is in the posterior aspects of deltoid. He has mild numbness over the posterior aspect of the right shoulder. Otherwise, the exam shows 5/5 muscle strength except shoulder abduction, which is 2/5. He has intact and symmetric DTRs throughout. Passive range of motion of the shoulder is full. Hawkin's, internal rotation lag, and Neer's test failed to illicit typical pain in the right shoulder.

3. What is the differential diagnosis?

4. What diagnostic tests would you order?

An NCS in the right upper extremity was unremarkable, except for absence of the sensory nerve action potential of the lateral antebrachial cutaneous nerve on the right (normal on left). EMG showed 1+ fibrillation potentials and 1+ positive waves in the right deltoid, biceps, and supraspinatus/infraspinatus muscles, but otherwise all normal in the right upper extremity and the cervical paraspinals. MRIs of the cervical spine and brachial plexus are normal.

5. What is the localization of the lesion and the most likely diagnosis? What is the prognosis? Describe the treatment program.

He read that a vaccination can cause an autoimmune disease. He works as a nurse and took a mandatory flu vaccine 1 month prior to his illness. He has hired an attorney to sue the hospital, and that attorney subpoenas your expert testimony.

6. How should you testify?

7. Explain his diagnosis and treatment to him in lay terms.

Answers

1. Questions involve the time course/progression of symptoms; distribution of muscle weakness; presence of atrophy; distribution of sensory deficits; how the symptoms limit his daily functions; and any joint pain.

2. Physical exams include DTRs, manual muscle testing, sensory exam, and musculoskeletal exam of the shoulder including active and passive range of motions, impingement signs, and scapular winging. Examine the skin for a herpetic rash.

3. At this point, differentials include cervical radiculopathy, herpes zoster, brachial plexopathy, nerve impingement (such as axillary impingement at the quadrangular space) syndrome, and musculoskeletal pain, such as rotator cuff syndrome.

4. EMG/NCS should be done to further localize the lesion. MRI of the cervical spine or brachial plexus may be ordered pending the results of the electrodiagnostic testing.

5. The physical exam and EMG/NCS are suggestive of the right brachial plexopathy, primarily upper trunk lesion. Given the acute history of shoulder pain, lack of trauma, or space-occupying lesion, the most likely diagnosis in this case is an inflammatory brachial plexopathy (Parsonage–Turner syndrome) in the right shoulder. About 89% of all the patients will eventually recover by the third year. Corticosteroids and IVIG are the initial treatment. Pain can be controlled with pregabalin or duloxetine. There are two aspects of rehab treatment in this case. First, functional deficits should be identified and addressed in PM&R clinic. For example, if he cannot reach out to a cabinet due to weakness in the right shoulder, one can consider training compensatory muscles with PT or getting a brace with OT or modifying his home environment. Second, a therapeutic exercise should be prescribed. There is some evidence that peripheral nerve regeneration is facilitated if a target muscle is stimulated. Therefore, exercising or electrical stimulation of the affected muscle can theoretically facilitate the recovery, and a physiatrist should be able to prescribe therapeutic exercise for the patient.

6. In testifying, research the facts ahead of time and limit your testimony to the scientific evidence, not your personal opinions. About 15% of Parsonage–Turner patients have a history of preceding vaccines, but 25% have a history of preceding viral illness. Parsonage–Turner is relatively common (reported incidence of 1.6/10,000 people). Given the low probability that an individual will become ill after a vaccine, the potential benefits of most vaccines outweigh any potential risks of developing autoimmune responses.

7. You need to use eighth-grade-level language and elicit whether he understands what you have explained. This is an inflammation of a nerve structure

called the brachial plexus. We do not know exactly how and why this happens, but it is thought that your own immune system is responsible for such inflammation. However, the good news is that it will slowly recover over time. Typically about 90% of patients will fully recover by the third year. In the meantime, it is important to continue exercising the shoulder muscle to facilitate the nerve recovery.

BIBLIOGRAPHY

Amato AA, Russell JA. Cervical and thoracic radiculopathies, brachial plexopathies, and mononeuropathies of the arm. In: Amato AA, Russell JA, eds. *Neuromuscular Disorder*. McGraw-Hill; 2008:chap 21.

Feinberg JH, Radecki J. Parsonage turner syndrome. *HSS J*. 2010;6(2):199–205. https://doi.org/10.1007/s11420-010-9176-x

Tsairis P, Dyck PJ, Mulder DW. Natural history of brachial plexus neuropathy. Report on 99 patients. *Arch Neurol*. August 1972;27(2):109–117. https://doi.org/10.1001/archneur.1972.00490140013004. PMID: 4339239.

van Alfen N, van Engelen BG. The clinical spectrum of neuralgic amyotrophy in 246 cases. *Brain*. February 2006;129 (Pt 2):438–450. https://doi.org/10.1093/brain/awh722. Epub 2005 Dec 21. PMID: 16371410.

10 Pain Rehabilitation

Andrew Nava

A 54-year-old woman presents in the clinic with epigastric pain, bloating, no nausea and vomiting, worsening pain with eating, and a new diagnosis of pancreatic cancer.

Questions

1. What more do you want to know about the patient's history, comorbidities, and social situation? Please tell me why you are asking for these specifics.

2. How would you go about performing a physical exam on this patient? Inspection, palpation of the abdomen and thoracic spine. Why are these maneuvers/exam components important?

She has 8/10 epigastric pain with radiation to the mid-back. It interferes with sleep, and she has been unable to work. Abdominal exam reveals mild guarding and no distension. She denies constipation or diarrhea and has no back pain or tenderness.

3. What is the differential diagnosis for this patient? Tell me the most likely diagnosis and why.

4. What diagnostic test or tests would you order and why?

Abdominal plain films and CT scan of the abdomen are unremarkable. MRI thoracic spine is not available.

5. Outline the treatment plan. Please tell me the initial treatment and next steps if that fails.

Add a scenario that has complexities of psychosocial situations or ethical dilemma. Examples might include insurance coverage, patient autonomy, advocacy, legal issues, or quality improvement.

The patient has collected a large bag full of narcotic and pain medications over the last year of her fight with cancer. She wants you to take them because she does not want them around her house.

6. What do you do?

The patient's spouse is concerned about your recommendation to start the patient on opioid therapy due to negative stories in the news and social media. How do you address this?

7. Tell me in lay terms about . . . Or how would you resolve this conflict?

Answers

1. What is the character of her pain? How severe is it on an analog scale, and how does it interfere with her function? How are her bowel movements?

2. Inspection is important to rule out a cutaneous cause of the pain, such as herpes zoster. Palpation of the abdomen is important to rule out a visceral cause (e.g., mass, rupture, etc.). Palpation of the thoracic spine is important to rule out a spinal etiology, such as fracture or spondylolisthesis, that may be causing a radiculitis.

3. Abdominal/cancer pain, constipation, inflammatory bowel disease (IBD). Cancer pain is the most likely and serious.

4. Abdominal plain films (to rule out ileus) and abdominal CT scan (to assess disease recurrence). MRI T-spine could be ordered if she had spinal tenderness to rule out metastases.

5. The plan is for a short course of opioids followed by a celiac plexus block.

6. Opiate disposal is a difficult issue in most jurisdiction. Many departments of public health will accept discarded narcotics on a daily basis or during drug collection days. The physician and the pharmacy are generally prohibited from accepting them in most states. Disposal down the toilet should be discouraged for environmental concerns. In the meantime, the patient should lock them up in a safe.

7. Opioids are the most effective medications for visceral cancer pain. In this case, celiac nerve block may provide some relief, but may not always eliminate all pain. We will monitor for signs and symptoms of abuse, and do periodic drug screens and pill counts to assure compliance. In addition, the medication should always remain locked up to keep others from getting into it, especially if there are adolescents in the household.

BIBLIOGRAPHY

Arcidiacono PGG, Calori G, Carrara S, et al. Celiac plexus block for pancreatic cancer pain in adults. *Cochrane Database Syst Rev.* March 2011;2011(3):CD007519. https://doi.org/10.1002/14651858.CD007519.pub2

Nersesyan H, Slavin K. Current approach to cancer pain management: availability and implications of different treatment options. *Ther Clin Risk Manag.* June 2007;3(3):381–400. https://doi.org/10.1186/1746-160X-3-30

CASE 2

A 35-year-old man fractured his left distal radius and ulnar in a fall 6 weeks ago. Upon removing the cast, his hand is exquisitely swollen, painful, and tender.

Questions

1. What more do you want to know about the patient's history, comorbidities, and social situation? Please tell me why you are asking for these specifics.

2. How would you go about performing a physical exam on this patient? Why are these maneuvers/exam components important?

He has no relevant past medical history. He has diffuse allodynia and hyperalgesia in his hand. His hand is cool. There is hair loss and nail bed changes. He has flexion of his fingers and poor grip.

3. What is the differential diagnosis for this patient? Tell me the most likely diagnosis and why.

4. What diagnostic test or tests would you order and why?

Compartment pressures are normal. The patient could not tolerate an electromyography (EMG)/nerve conduction study (NCS). X-ray shows a well-healed fracture but diffuse osteopenia of the hand.

5. Outline the treatment plan. Please tell me the initial treatment and next steps if that fails.

The fall occurred at work. He is a short-order cook.

6. What obligations does his employer (or workers' compensation insurer) have in terms of his rehabilitation and compensation?

The patient demands opioids because he "can't take the pain anymore."

7. How do you respond to him?

CASE 2

Answers

1. How did the fracture occur? What is the character of the pain? Does he have involvement of any other joints? Does he have any significant past history? The Budapest criteria for complex regional pain syndrome (CRPS) require symptoms in three of the following four categories: sensory, vasomotor (cyanosis or erythema), sudomotor/edema, and motor (atrophy or loss of range of motion).

2. A focused musculoskeletal and neurologic exam of the hand and upper extremity should be performed. The contralateral hand and extremity should also be examined to note any asymmetries or discrepancies. The Budapest criteria must include signs in two of the four earlier categories.

3. Differential diagnosis includes compartment syndrome, nonunion, nerve injury, and CRPS. The patient meets the Budapest criteria.

4. Compartment pressures should be checked urgently. Electrodiagnostic testing can be helpful if tolerated. X-rays should be obtained to look at fracture healing as well as osteopenia, which can be seen in severe CRPS.

5. He likely has CRPS. A stellate ganglion block is the best initial treatment in acute onset upper limb CRPS. Neuropathic pain medicines such as gabapentin or serotonin–norepinephrine reuptake inhibitors (SNRIs) may help. Tricyclic antidepressants (TCAs) may also be helpful. The role of corticosteroids is unclear, but a short course might be tried. Physical or occupational hand therapy can include contrast baths, fluidotherapy, compression wraps, desensitization techniques, range of motion exercises, and strengthening as tolerated. Early return to activity is thought to be helpful.

6. The employer is responsible for providing not only medical treatments, but also comprehensive rehabilitation, including vocational services not typically covered by medical insurance. In addition, the employer must provide compensation until the patient can return to his old job. If the employee is unable to return to his previous job (permanent disability), then the employer must provide retraining for other work or pay a permanent disability reward based on his level of impairment and his previous income.

7. First, make sure he does not have active suicidal ideation. Explain to the patient that there are other options for his pain, including physical therapy, injections, and nonopioid medications. Explain that these treatments, when adhered to, may significantly reduce his pain, improve his function, and restore his quality of life over time. Opioids are a last resort if all else fails.

BIBLIOGRAPHY

Harden RN, Bruehl S, Perez RS, et al. Validation of proposed diagnostic criteria (the "Budapest Criteria") for complex regional pain syndrome. *Pain.* 2010;150:268–274. https://doi.org/10.1016/j.pain.2010.04.030

Shin H, Rose J, Halle S, et al. Complex regional pain syndrome: a narrative review for the practising clinician. *Br J Anaesth.* August 2019;123(2):e424–e433. https://doi.org/10.1016/j.bja.2019.03.030

CASE 3

A 25-year-old woman presents with a 2-month history of pain in the neck, shoulders, back, and hips. She has no significant past medical history and has had no trauma.

Questions

1. What more do you want to know about the patient's history, comorbidities, and social situation? Please tell me why you are asking for these specifics.

2. How would you go about performing a physical exam on this patient?

She has generalized achy pain. There are no radicular symptoms and no joint swelling. Pain interrupts her sleep. She gets no exercise.

3. What is the differential diagnosis for this patient? Tell me the most likely diagnosis and why.

4. What diagnostic test or tests would you order and why?

She has no evidence of inflammatory arthritis on her labs. She has a normal MRI of the brain and cervical spine.

5. Outline the treatment plan. Please tell me the initial treatment and next steps if that fails.

She tells you she wants to apply for Social Security disability. How should you respond?

6. How should you respond?

She states that exercise just makes her worse.

7. Explain to the patient the importance of exercise for this diagnosis?

Answers

1. You should question the patient about the character of the pain, exacerbating and relieving factors, radiation, arthralgias, numbness, weakness, and bowel and bladder symptoms. You should ask about sleep, exercise, and vocational and avocational interests. You should ask about past medical and family history.

2. Joints should be examined for synovitis and range of motion. A spine exam including Hoffman's and Spurling's tests should be performed. A thorough neurologic exam should include a check of motor and sensory impairments, reflexes, and balance. A tender point exam should be performed.

3. The differential diagnosis for diffuse axial pain in a young person includes cervical spine disease, Arnold Chiari malformation, myositis, inflammatory arthritis, multiple sclerosis, and fibromyalgia (FM). FM is a diagnosis of exclusion, but may be the most likely in this case.

4. Testing should include an autoimmune profile, creatine kinase (CK), and MRI of the c-spine and brain.

5. She likely has FM. Treatment focuses on improving sleep and gradual increase in exercise. Medications effective for FM include pregabalin, gabapentin, and SNRIs. The combination of pregabalin and duloxetine has been shown to be more effective than either of them alone. Secondary medications include TCAs and cyclobenzaprine. Sleep medication, particularly over-the-counter agents such as melatonin or diphenhydramine, may be helpful. Opioids and nonsteroidal anti-inflammatory drugs (NSAIDs) are generally not effective for FM and should be avoided. List the most likely and other relevant possibilities.

6. Social Security Disability has a very high threshold for qualification. She would need to demonstrate that she is unable to perform any work irrespective of occupation. Most people with FM are able to work at least sedentary jobs. She would likely get rejected.

7. First, explain the scientific evidence for exercise in FM in lay terms. Behavioral interviewing would be helpful. Engage her in readiness for change, ask about barriers to exercise, and explain how she could overcome these barriers.

BIBLIOGRAPHY

Clauw DJ. Fibromyalgia: a clinical review. *JAMA.* 2014;311(15):1547–1555. https://doi.org/10.1001/jama.2014.3266

Davies M, Ward C, Singh J. Fibromyalgia. https://now.aapmr.org/fibromyalgia. March 27, 2017.

Wolfe F, Walitt B, Perrot S, et al. Fibromyalgia diagnosis and biased assessment: sex, prevalence and bias. *PLOS ONE.* 2018;13(9):e02037551. https://doi.org/10.1371/journal.pone.0203755

11 Pediatric Rehabilitation

Sarah A. Korth

A 15-month-old child is brought to the pediatrician's office for evaluation due to concern about developmental delay.

Questions

1. What more do you want to know about the patient's history, comorbidities, and social situation? Please tell me why you are asking for these specifics.

2. How would you go about performing a physical exam on this patient? Why are these maneuvers/exam components important?

Records brought to the visit reveal the child was adopted from China at the age of 12 months. Prenatal and birth history are not available and medical/developmental information is limited. The mom does know the child was born full term. The child lived in an orphanage until adoption. Mom reports the child is not yet walking but is beginning to pull to stand. The child favors the right hand, which was noted at the orphanage.

Physical exam findings include normal growth parameters, including head circumference. He has decreased functional use of the left upper extremity compared to the right. Active movement of the wrists are noted to have flexion and extension with reaching. At rest, the left forearm is more pronated than the right and the left hand tends to remain closed with thumb tucked while right hand remains relaxed and open. Passively, range is full. Left lower extremity with decreased passive range at the ankle and mild tightness of the hamstring is noted, as well as two beats of clonus at the ankle. The child is able to maintain sitting balance independently and can pull to sit, typically using the right extremity. When placed in supported standing, the right foot is flat and the left is plantar flexed at initial foot contact but can relax to foot flat. The child speaks at least five to 10 words in Chinese and says three to four words in English.

3. What is the differential diagnosis for this patient? Tell me the most likely diagnosis and why.

4. What diagnostic test or tests would you order and why?

MRI reveals a middle cerebral artery infarction that is likely intrauterine or perinatal.

5. Outline the treatment plan.

The mother tells you she cannot afford the co-payments on the child's rehabilitation therapies.

6. What options does she have?

As you are finishing the visit, the mother asks, "Will my child walk and be normal like other kids?"

7. What is your response to this mother?

Answers

1. Information regarding prenatal, birth, and developmental history should be elicited, including sitting, standing, holding onto a table or with assistance, cruising, grasp abilities of the hands, and what activities can be done with each hand/arm. Information should be obtained about speech, oral motor skills, and eating. Any known medical history, including trauma, should be obtained. Are there vision or hearing issues? History of seizures? Any imaging or other evaluations that have been completed?

2. Obtain height, weight, and head circumference, which can alert to need for further evaluation that may include brain structure and growth, genetic testing, and nutritional assessments. Physical exam should include passive and active range of motion (ROM) of major joints in upper and lower limbs, noting contractures and weakness. Tone in neck, trunk, and all limbs should be assessed, including clonus. Make particular note of any asymmetry on physical exam. Evaluate for developmental milestones attained, including grasp, sitting, and pulling to stand, and assess mobility.

3. Based on history and physical examination, this child is not meeting developmental milestones and has abnormalities in motor function in hemiplegic pattern; left hemiplegic cerebral palsy is the most likely diagnosis. "Cerebral palsy" refers to disorders of the development of movement and posture, causing activity limitation, that are attributed to *nonprogressive* disturbances that occurred in the developing fetal or infant brain.

4. MRI of the brain, in conjunction with the clinical history, may determine etiology in many children with cerebral palsy, including ischemic stroke and cerebral dysgenesis. MRI may also rule out potentially treatable causes of motor impairments, such as tumor or hydrocephalus. MRIs do little to guide management of motor impairments in cerebral palsy.

5. Constraint-induced movement therapy (CIMT) should be recommended in this child to facilitate spontaneous use of the left upper extremity, as well as functional finger movements. Physical therapy should be recommended to facilitate gross motor skills, including standing and ambulation. As the child starts to do more weight-bearing and ambulation, foot and ankle position should be monitored to determine the need for bracing to facilitate a normal gait pattern. Activities to encourage muscle strengthening and functional use are incorporated into play skills.

6. The child may be eligible for therapy in preschool.

7. Children with hemiplegia due to perinatal ischemic stroke are typically independent ambulators and walk by age 2, if not sooner. Most kids develop functional use of the affected hand but for some fine motor skills may be impaired. Most have normal intelligence and participate in a regular school program and

typical recreational activities. If upper extremity weakness causes functional impairments, accommodations can be made.

BIBLIOGRAPHY

Ashwal S, Russman BS, Blasco PA, et al. Practice parameter: diagnostic assessment of the child with cerebral palsy: report of the quality standards subcommittee of the American academy of neurology and the practice committee of the child neurology society. *Neurology.* 2004;62(6):851–863. https://doi.org/10.1212/01.WNL.0000117981.35364.1B

Kitai Y, Haginoya K, Hirai S, et al. Outcome of hemiplegic cerebral palsy born at term depends on its etiology. *Brain Dev.* March 2016;38(3):267–273. https://doi.org/10.1016/j.braindev.2015.09.007

Rosenbaum P, Dan B, Leviton A, et al. Proposed definition and classification of cerebral palsy, April 2005. *Dev Med Child Neurol.* 2005;47:571–576. https://doi.org/10.1017/S001216220500112X

Shin M, Kim H. Cerebral palsy. https://now.aapmr.org/cerebral-palsy. April 17, 2017. Accessed January 17, 2021.

CASE 2

A 6-year-old girl is admitted to a pediatric rehabilitation unit 3 months following a severe traumatic brain injury (TBI). The initial Glasgow Coma Scale score was 5 with prolonged loss of consciousness.

Questions

1. What more do you want to know about the patient's history and social situation? Please tell me why you are asking for these specifics.

2. How would you go about performing a physical exam on this patient? Why are these maneuvers/exam components important?

The child was in a coma for 7 days. She reports no pain. She is verbal but oriented to person only. She has no hemiparesis.

3. How does the child's prognosis compare to that of a teenager or young adult with the same injury?

4. What cognitive impairments would you screen for over the course of her recovery?

The patient has progressed to a Rancho 4/5 level and is becoming agitated on the unit. She has kicked and bitten staff members.

5. What strategies can be used to help manage the agitation, both non-medication and medication? What are the risks/side effects associated with medication use?

The patient has been in inpatient rehabilitation for 3 weeks and is no longer agitated, but safety and learning concerns persist due to inattention and short-term memory problems.

6. What special learning considerations exist for the school-aged child with a TBI over time? How might school reintegration be facilitated?

The parents of the child approach you to express their concerns about managing their child's needs when she returns home and goes back to school. They mention that stressors have been "through the roof" since the accident, with both parents having to miss work during the hospital stay, challenges with their employers, financial strain, as well as regression of behaviors in their 5-year-old son, who has been acting out much more.

7. After you reviewed the earlier school reintegration plans, how would you address the parents' concerns with them in lay terms?

Answers

1. Important history to obtain includes:
   a. Rancho level
   b. Duration of coma
   c. Ability to communicate
   d. Presence of pain
   e. Social history (note that family dysfunction and stress tend to increase following pediatric brain injury and the child's social situation should remain an important focus throughout the recovery process)

2. Important components of examination include:
   a. Assessment for pain (care team should be vigilant to the surfacing of overlooked injuries, such as level of alertness changes and localizing pain, as well as new secondary pathologies that may begin to arise, such as heterotopic ossification)
   b. Muscle strength
   c. Presence of contractures
   d. Cognitive exam
   e. Sensation
   f. Skin integrity
   g. Functional assessment

3. Children with a brain injury are at increased risk for negative outcomes compared to adults. Injury during early childhood and elementary school may cause worse outcomes compared to injury as teenagers. When children are injured at a younger age, it can impair their ability to gain the skills needed for later development. Milestones may not be reached that would allow the child to gain new skills.

4. Cognitive impairments in pediatric TBI commonly affect:
   a. Arousal and attention
   b. Memory
   c. Behaviors
   d. Communication
   e. Executive function
   f. Social skills

5. Strategies may include environmental changes as well as medications.
   a. Environmental strategies: Avoid overstimulation, maintain a quiet environment, have consistent staff treat the patient, provide frequent reassurance, and evaluate the impact of visitors and therapy, limiting them if causing agitation. Promote adequate sleep. Avoid use of restraints.

b. Pharmacological strategies: Literature involving pediatric patients is limited.

i. Benzodiazepines may be utilized but are not considered a good long-term solution. They may cause sedation and decreased concentration.

ii. Beta-blockers may be used until the intensity of agitation decreases. Side effects include bradycardia, orthostatic hypotension, and fatigue.

iii. Anticonvulsants' side effects may include negative effects on cognitive and motor function.

iv. Antipsychotics: Adult studies have shown slow cognitive improvement or decreased cognitive return. The side effect list is long and can include weight gain, extrapyramidal symptoms, and neuroleptic malignant syndrome.

6. School reintegration is an important goal for the school-age child. As school progresses, demands increase in complexity. For children post-TBI who have difficulty with memory and executive functioning, the increased complexity of demands becomes more difficult to manage and they may fall behind their peers. The Individuals with Disabilities Education Act (IDEA) included TBI as an eligible condition for educational assistance within the public school system in the form of Individual Educational Plans (IEPs) that led to a shift from focus on the academic performance alone to the child's global functioning, including motor, attention, and executive functioning. There should be a team approach to the creation and ongoing management of the IEP involving the family, the school, and the rehabilitation team. The preparation of the initial IEP should begin while the child is still admitted to inpatient rehabilitation to facilitate a smooth transition into the school environment.

7. A brain injury in a child affects the entire family unit. The impact may include emotional and financial stressors and shifts in responsibilities to adapt to the changes. Preinjury family functioning has also been demonstrated to have an impact on the long-term outcome of the child with an acquired brain injury. Proactive, comprehensive services are important not only for the child but for the entire family. Caregivers should be reassured early in the course that rehabilitation is a continuum of care and does not stop at the time of discharge. Early and continued supportive child and family counseling and education about TBI and its consequences should be implemented. Peer support and medical play can be helpful to siblings as well as to patients. Early contact with caregivers' employers and exploration of alternative funding sources as needed by the rehabilitation team can be of substantial benefit. Continued rehabilitation team involvement in coordination of medical- and education-based services facilitates effective reintegration into the home and community.

BIBLIOGRAPHY

Backeljauw B, Kurowski B. Interventions for attention problems after pediatric traumatic brain injury: what is the evidence? *PM&R*. 2014;6:814–824. https://doi.org/10.1016/j.pmrj.2014.04.004

Cole W, Paulos S, Cole C, et al. A review of family intervention guidelines for pediatric acquired brain injuries. *Dev Disabil Res Rev*. 2009;15:159–166. https://doi.org/10.1002/ddrr.58

Krach L, Gormley M, Ward M. Traumatic brain injury. In: Alexander M, Matthews D, eds. *Pediatric Rehabilitation: Principles and Practice*. Demos Medical Publishing; 2015:chap 17.

Pangilinan P, Giacoletti-Argento A, Shellhaas R, et al. Neuropharmacology in pediatric brain injury: a review. *PM&R*. 2010;2:1127–1140. https://doi.org/10.1016/j.pmrj.2010.07.007

Ponsford J, Janzen S, McIntyre A, et al. INCOG recommendations for management of cognition following traumatic brain injury, Part 1: posttraumatic amnesia/delirium. *J Head Trauma Rehabil.* 2014;29(4):307–320. https://doi.org/10.1097/HTR.0000000000000074

Rauh M, Aralis H, Melcer T, et al. Effect of traumatic brain injury among US service members with amputation. *JRRD.* 2013;50:161–172. https://doi.org/10.1682/JRRD.2011.11.0212

Suskauer S, Trovato M. Update on pharmaceutical intervention for disorders of consciousness and agitation after traumatic brain injury in children. *PM&R.* 2013;5:142–147. https://doi.org/10.1016/j.pmrj.2012.08.021

An 11-year-old gymnast sees you for lower back pain. She is very active in her sport and participates in local and regional competitions.

Questions

1. What more do you want to know about the patient's history? Please tell me why you are asking for these specifics.

2. How would you go about performing a physical exam on this patient? Why are these maneuvers/exam components important?

Pain is relatively sharp and worse with extension. On examination, she has tightness of her hamstrings and quads. There is localized tenderness in the left upper lumbar paraspinal musculature. Pain does not radiate into the lower limbs and strength is normal.

3. What is the differential diagnosis for this patient? Tell me the most likely diagnosis and why.

4. What diagnostic test or tests would you order and why? If an x-ray is ordered, what views would you order and why?

Lumbar x-ray (anteroposterior [AP] and lateral only) shows no abnormalities. MRI is normal. What is your next step? What instructions will you give to the patient?

5. Outline the treatment plan. Please tell me the initial treatment and next steps if that fails.

The CT in Figure 11.1 shows a bilateral L5 pars low-grade stress fracture.

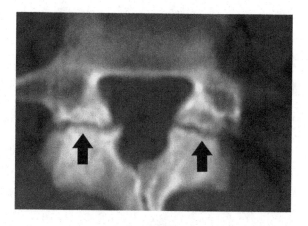

Figure 11.1 CT spondylolysis.

When you share this with the patient and family, they express concern because she has an important competition coming up and would like to know how soon she can return to practice. They tell you "she is tough and can probably push through it".

6. How would you respond?

7. In lay terms, explain the diagnosis to the patient and parents.

Answers

1. It is critical to assess the onset and duration of pain and if there were any acute trauma, as well as exacerbating or remitting factors. A lower limb neurologic examination should be completed.

2. Physical examination should include inspection and palpation of spinous processes and paraspinal musculature for tenderness and step off; thoraco-lumbo-sacral spine ROM; bilateral lower limb passive and active ROM; lower limb strength, sensory, and reflex testing; and observation of gait.

3. Differential diagnosis includes spondylolysis, spondylolisthesis, lumbar strain, tumor, and infection.

4. Tests include lumbar spine x-ray with AP, lateral, and oblique views and lumbar spine MRI.

5. The next step is minimization of aggravating activities, as well as physical therapy directed at lower limb flexibility, core strengthening, and modalities for pain. Instructions include temporary removal from extension-based activities (removal from sport). If pain does not improve, MRI should be ordered (if not already completed) and a bone scan with single-photon emission computed tomography (SPECT), as the SPECT scan shows uptake at the bilateral L5 pars interarticularis, which can be missed on MRI. You may then order a thin cut CT through the area of uptake to evaluate for pars stress fracture. If pain persists after therapy, next step is Boston bracing for 3 months with continued follow-up; spine surgery if the fracture progresses.

6. This is a very serious injury that often results in major surgery should it progress. It would probably be better if she pursued a noncontact sport. She certainly should not return to gymnastics until the pars fracture is healed.

7. This should be done in eighth-grade language. Her backbone is cracked and may slip out of place.

BIBLIOGRAPHY

Klein G, Mehlman CT, McCarty M. Nonoperative treatment of spondylolysis and grade I spondylolisthesis in children and young adults: a meta-analysis of observational studies. *J Pediatr Orthop.* 2009;29(2):146–156. https://doi.org/10.1097/BPO.0b013e3181977fc5

Leonidou A, Lepetsos P, Pagkalos J, et al. Treatment for spondylolysis and spondylolisthesis in children. *J Orthop Surg.* 2015;23(3):379–382. https://doi.org/10.1177/230949901502300326

CASE 4

A 10-year-old female presents to your office with her mother. The mother states that the patient was undergoing a routine physical examination by her family doctor for sports participation when she was found to have scoliosis. She was then referred to you for management.

Questions

1. What more do you want to know about the patient's history? Please tell me why you are asking for these specifics.

2. Taking into consideration the referring diagnosis, what are the key components of her physical examination? Why are these maneuvers/exam components important?

She does not complain of any neurologic symptoms, has a normal birth history and childhood, and has no relevant family history. On exam, you find no dysmorphic anatomy or any signs of congenital disease. She is neurologically intact with normal strength, sensation, and reflexes. Her spine has a rightward thoracolumbar curve, and there is protrusion of the right rib cage and scapula.

3. What is the differential diagnosis for this patient? Tell me the most likely diagnosis and why.

4. What diagnostic test or tests would you order and why?

The radiographs show a 20-degree curvature.

5. Outline your management plan.

The patient expresses concern about her appearance.

6. How can this be addressed?

The mother asks why her daughter has a curved spine and if her daughter is going to need surgery. She then asks if her daughter will need a back brace or any additional treatments.

7. How would you respond?

CASE 4

Answers

1. Are there any pain or neurologic symptoms present (i.e., numbness, tingling, or weakness)? What is the patient's birth and pediatric milestone history (including growth)? Is there a family history of scoliosis or neuromuscular disease?

2. Key components include inspection/observation (any dysmorphic features or other signs of neuromuscular disorders; that is, café-au-lait spots, dimpling of skin or tuft of hair over low back, long fingers or chest deformities); neurologic exam of cranial nerves and limbs (sensation, reflexes, and strength); musculoskeletal exam (inspection/palpation of spine and limbs, ROM of spine, chest expansion, gait analysis).

3. Differential diagnosis includes congenital, neuromuscular, or idiopathic scoliosis.

4. Diagnostic tests include standing upright, plain radiographs of the spine (cervical, thoracic, and lumbar to measure degree of scoliosis), and pelvic radiograph (to measure Risser grade and better predict bone growth potential).

5. If the curvature is <30 degrees, management is conservative with repeat x-rays in 1 year.

6. Peer counseling can be beneficial if you have a support group in your area. Alternatively, psychological counseling may be needed, particularly if depressive symptoms develop.

7. This is a great opportunity for patient and parent education regarding the patient's condition. There should be a discussion about the types of scoliosis (congenital, neuromuscular, and idiopathic), about how the most common cause is idiopathic, and how most cases do not require surgery. Also, assure the parent that you will refer the patient to the appropriate surgical specialist if needed. Clarity of explanation and ability to give information in a compassionate, thoughtful, and caring manner are necessary. Whether or not the patient will require bracing or any further treatment will be based on the degree of curvature, the potential for future growth, and the progression of the scoliotic curve over time. This is an opportunity to again educate the patient and parent in a clear, compassionate, and thoughtful manner.

BIBLIOGRAPHY

El-Hawary R, Chukwunyerenwa C. Update on evaluation and treatment of scoliosis. *Pediatr Clin North Am.* 2014;61(6):1223–1241. https://doi.org/10.1016/j.pcl.2014.08.007

Horne JP, Flannery R, Usman S. Adolescent idiopathic scoliosis: diagnosis and management. *Am Fam Physician.* 2014;89(3):193–198.

CASE 5

A 14-year-old female with a sacral-level myelomeningocele who has not required an assistive device on prior evaluations presents to the Multidisciplinary Spina Bifida Clinic today using Lofstrand crutches.

Questions

1. What more do you want to know about the patient's history? Please tell me why you are asking for these specifics.

2. How would you go about performing a physical exam on this patient? Why are these maneuvers/exam components important?

She was last seen in this Multidisciplinary Spina Bifida Clinic 2 years ago. Her symptoms began about 10 months ago. She appears uncomfortable and complains of "tingly" feelings in her feet and increased fatigue. Her weakness is localized to the lower extremities. She reports that her back aches, especially after a busy day at school. She also states that her feet "look different." No fevers, headaches, diplopia, emesis, or lethargy are reported. She does have shunted hydrocephalus that has never required a revision. Vital signs are normal. She has no cranial nerve deficits. Vocal quality and volume are unchanged. Examination of the lower extremities shows left knee flexion is weaker than right. Foot inversion is weak on both sides. There is a calcaneovalgus appearance of the foot.

3. What is the differential diagnosis for her weakness? Tell me the most likely diagnosis and why.

4. What diagnostic test or tests would you order and why?

Her MRI of the spine shows tethering of the cord at T11 to L1.

5. Outline the treatment plan.

The reason she has not seen you in 2 years is that she missed her 6-month interval appointments in the spina bifida clinic.

6. How would you address this with the patient and her family?

7. Explain tethering of the spinal cord in lay terms to the patient and her family.

CASE 5

Answers

1. Does she have shunted hydrocephalus? Does she have headaches, lethargy, diplopia, or emesis? Any changes in vocal quality or swallowing function? Any back pain, new numbness, or tingling? Has the family noticed any change in foot position/appearance compared to the past? Is there a change in her bladder and/or bowel function/patterns? Has she gained weight? Any injuries or surgeries?

2. Her neuromusculoskeletal exam should include a cranial nerve exam; a detailed assessment of her lower limbs, including visual inspection of her feet, passive range of motion (PROM) of all major joints in lower limbs, sensation testing, and manual motor testing; as well as careful observation of her gait.

3. Differential diagnosis includes tethered cord, shunt malfunction, syringomyelia, compressive bone abnormalities, weakness secondary to weight gain, and deconditioning. Tethered cord is most likely.

4. CT or MRI of the head is required to evaluate for obstructive hydrocephalus. MRI of the spine is also warranted to evaluate for tethered cord and syringomyelia given the loss of muscle strength and new sensory symptoms in lower legs and feet. Other studies could include spine x-rays or spine CT to look for bony abnormalities and to assess for scoliosis. Manual muscle testing and urodynamic testing should also be performed to document any changes and to provide a presurgical baseline.

5. Referral should be made to a neurosurgeon. Since almost all patients with spina bifida have some evidence of tethering on MRI, clinical judgment that includes clear evidence of deterioration in function is required before surgical untethering. All previous neuroimaging studies should be made available to the neurosurgeon. Symptomatic tethering can occur at any time throughout life.

6. Deterioration of function is more difficult to reverse the longer the tethering is untreated. It is important not to miss scheduled appointments to the Spina Bifida Program. One should not be judgmental and should ask why the patient missed the appointments. Did the patient refuse? Did the family lose medical insurance? Was transportation a problem?

7. In eighth-grade language, explain that the spinal cord has become tangled/caught. Treatment is usually surgical. Be careful not to be too scary in your language, and emphasize that this is treatable when caught early.

BIBLIOGRAPHY

Bui CJ, Tubbs RS, Oakes WJ. Tethered cord syndrome in children: a review. *Neurosurg Focus.* 2007;23(2):1–9. https://doi.org/10.3171/FOC-07/08/E2

Dicianno BE, Kurowski BG, Yang JMJ, et al. Rehabilitation and medical management of the adult with spina bifida. *Am J Phys Med Rehabil.* 2008;87:1026–1050. https://doi.org/10.1097/PHM.0b013e31818de070

Spina Bifida Association. Guidelines for the care of people with Spina Bifida. 2018. http://www.spinabifidaassociation.org/guidelines/

CASE 6

A 5-year-old boy is brought to a pediatric physical medicine and rehabilitation (PM&R) clinic. His mother reports he was typically developing until 1 year ago, when he began having a harder time walking.

Questions

1. What more do you want to know about the patient's history, comorbidities, and social situation? Please tell me why you are asking for these specifics.

2. How would you go about performing a physical exam on this patient? Why are these maneuvers/exam components important?

The mother says the patient uses his hands to stand up from the ground. The decline in strength started about 1 year ago. The mother was adopted and does not know if anyone in her family had neurological disorders. The boy's sister is 2 years older than he is and healthy.

3. What is the differential diagnosis for this patient?

4. What diagnostic test or tests would you order and why?

An electrodiagnostic study showed normal sensory conduction results, but electromyography (EMG) shows small units with early recruitment patterns in proximal muscles. A muscle biopsy showed many atrophic myofibers with extensive necrosis and intermysial fibrosis. A further genetic workup reveals a mutation in the dystrophin gene.

5. What is the prognosis? Outline the medical and rehabilitative treatment plan. Please tell me the initial treatment and next steps if that fails.

Five years later, the patient comes back to your clinic and his mother is concerned about his poor academic performance. Per his mother, he was an A student, but since the new semester, he appears tired all the time and is seen sleeping during the class.

6. What is your approach to this problem?

Fifteen years later, the patient comes back to your clinic after having fallen off from a bed during transfer. He is complaining of chest pain. He is currently living in a group home and is dependent with all aspects of activities of daily living. On inspection, there are multiple bruises ion the chest and trunk, and some of them appear to be old.

7. What would you do?

Answers

1. Questions include pregnancy, birth, and developmental histories; time course/progression of symptoms; presence and distribution of sensory symptoms; pattern of muscle weakness; presence of musculoskeletal pain; and family history.

2. Items to evaluate include tone, deep tendon reflexes, strength and sensory exams, gait analysis, cardiac auscultation (to rule out murmur), and general morphological inspection.

3. Differential diagnosis include muscular dystrophy, spinal muscular atrophy, congenital myopathy, juvenile dermatomyositis, and mitochondrial myopathy.

4. Workup includes nerve conduction studies (NCS) and EMG, muscle biopsy, and genetic workup (including evaluation of dystrophin gene).

5. This is Duchenne muscular dystrophy, which is a progressive, fatal disease. He will likely be wheelchair-dependent during his teenage years, and his expected life span is 20 to 30 years. Given the progressive nature of the disease, early rehabilitative intervention is important. For example, a rollator can be considered for ambulation at this stage, but as he loses his ability to walk, a motorized wheelchair should be considered. Bracing is also needed to prevent scoliosis. In addition, he can be started on prednisone to delay the progression of motor weakness after discussion with his family regarding potential benefits and risks.

6. Careful physical examination and medication history is important. Daytime narcolepsy is an early sign of respiratory distress due to reduced vital capacity, and history of sleep apnea should be obtained. If needed, pulmonary function tests should be considered. Psychosocial aspects of his school life should be examined, as he is undergoing adolescence with severe disability. Symptoms of depression, his social life with peers, and the possibility of bullying should be addressed.

7. Obtain histories from caretakers and family members. Evaluate vital signs and changes in body mass index (BMI). Physical exam of the chest, including inspection, palpation, and auscultation, is the first step to rule out any life-threatening conditions. Evaluate patient thoroughly for signs/symptoms of neglect or abuse. If it appears that he has been neglected or abused at the group home, Adult Protective Services should be contacted and family and facility made aware.

BIBLIOGRAPHY

Amato AA, Russell JA. Muscular dystrophies. In: Amato AA, Russell JA, eds. *Neuromuscular disorders.* McGraw-Hill; 2008:chap 24.

Bushby K, Finkel R, Birnkrant DJ, et al. Diagnosis and management of Duchenne muscular dystrophy, part 1: diagnosis and pharmacological and psychosocial management. *Lancet Neurol.* 2010;9(1):77–93. https://doi.org/10.1016/S1474-4422(09)70271-6

Kellogg ND, Committee on Child Abuse and Neglect, American Academy of Pediatrics. Evaluation of suspected child physical abuse. *Peds.* 2007;119(6):1232–1241. https://doi.org/10.1542/peds.2007-0883

CASE 7

A 5-year-old boy is brought into the office by his father, who states that the child "has hardly been able to walk" for the last couple of days.

Questions

1. What more do you want to know about the patient's history and comorbidities? Describe why you are asking for these specifics.

2. How would you go about performing a physical exam on this patient? Why are these maneuvers/exam components important?

The boy was in his normal state of health until 2 days ago, when he developed right-sided hip pain and a limp. He had a sore throat a few weeks prior. The father notes that he gave the boy ibuprofen for discomfort this morning, which seemed to help a small amount. He also mentions he took the boy's temperature a couple of hours later, and it was 100°F. Weight-bearing or moving the hip exacerbates the pain, while sitting and lying make it better. He has otherwise been healthy with no weight loss, changes in appetite, or changes in overall energy level. His father denies any known trauma but admits the boy roughhouses with his older brother regularly. He is well-appearing, blood pressure (BP) is normal, and he has slight tachycardia as well as a temporal temperature of 101°F. You observe the boy walk into the room with an antalgic gait, limiting weight-bearing on the right leg. On inspection, muscle bulk appears normal and symmetric. On PROM, there is limitation in right hip abduction and internal rotation and the boy guards the right hip when examiner moves it, but the remainder of the ROM is normal. His strength testing is normal for age throughout, but right hip strength testing is limited due to pain. His reflexes are normal and he has down-going toes to the Babinski test bilaterally. On skin evaluation, there are no rashes or localized edema, erythema, or warmth of either hip or knee.

3. What is the differential diagnosis for this patient? Tell me the most likely diagnosis and why.

4. What are your next steps and what studies do you recommend?

Bloodwork and hip x-ray were completed and you review the results, noting that the white blood cell count (WBC) is slightly elevated, but erythrocyte sedimentation rate (ESR) and C-reactive protein (CRP) are within normal limits. The hip x-ray appears normal.

5. Outline the treatment plan. Please tell me initial treatment and next steps if that fails.

The father tells you that there was debate between the doctors in the ED on whether to complete a hip x-ray, a hip ultrasound (US), or an MRI with sedation. He ponders why all of these diagnostic tests were not performed if they each add additional information. He also admits, however, that he did not push further for these tests as he was feeling some time pressure as a result of previously planned evening obligations. The father's comment makes you think more about all the factors that go into diagnostic workup and treatment planning.

6. Describe several steps that are essential to a risk-benefit analysis when determining a diagnostic or treatment plan in similar situations.

The father calls your office from the ED at the end of the day before you have left for the weekend and asks for a plan for follow-up office visit. He mentions he was planning to leave the ED as he does not have time to wait any longer for the hip US. He states that the bloodwork and the x-ray were normal, so the problem is unlikely to be an infection in his son's hip. He plans to give the boy ibuprofen for comfort when he gets home. He states he will bring him back next week if it gets worse.

7. How might you explain the importance of the situation to the father?

Answers

1. History should include constitutional symptoms, including fever, changes in energy level, appetite, and weight, which give clues to systemic processes. It is important to focus on details of the pain, including its onset, location, radiation, duration, quality, aggravating and alleviating factors, and any associated weaknesses. A history of recent upper respiratory illnesses and trauma should be discussed, as well as a past medical and surgical history review. These questions help with development of a differential diagnosis to guide subsequent workup.

2. The physical exam should include a detailed bilateral lower limb evaluation, including observation for muscle bulk and symmetry, skin inspection for localized erythema and palpation for warmth around joints, PROM, and pain with joint movement. Limited internal rotation and abduction of the hip can be associated with many common hip pathologies in pediatrics, and severity of pain with PROM and with weight-bearing can give important clues as to etiology. Gait analysis should be completed with attention to the presence of antalgic or Trendelenburg gait, which can be related to pain in the hip or in the gluteus medius muscle.

3. a. Differential diagnosis: A differential diagnosis for pediatric atraumatic hip pain and limp should include septic arthritis of the hip (SA), acute transient synovitis (ATS), Legg-Calve-Perthes Disease (LCP), and slipped capital femoral epiphysis (SCFE). Some of the differences are summarized in the following table.

	SA	ATS	LCP	SCFE
ETIOLOGY AND PATHOLOGY	– Etiology unclear, but can be associated with trauma or surgery, hematologic spread of infection, or spread from osteomyelitis of femoral head. – Purulent exudate rapidly destroys hyaline cartilage	– Etiology unclear (viral etiologies suspected)	– Avascular necrosis of proximal femur – Thought to be due to rapid bone growth with insufficient blood supply to meet demand	– Epiphysiolysis/ proximal femoral epiphysis separates at the growth plate
AGE OF ONSET	Usually <2 years old	3–6 years old	4–10 years old	9–15 years old

(Continued)

	SA	ATS	LCP	SCFE
RISK FACTORS	– M>F	– M>F – Recent URI – Recent trauma	– M>F	– M>F – Obesity – Blacks>Whites
HISTORY	– Onset: Rapid (days) – Unilateral pain	– Onset: Rapid (days) – Unilateral limp – Unilateral hip/groin pain – Healthy child, may have low-grade fever	– Onset: Weeks to months – Pain in unilateral hip/groin, radiates to medial thigh/knee	– Unilateral (25% bilateral) – Pain in hip/ groin, radiates to medial thigh/ knee
PHYSICAL EXAM	– Preferred resting position of hip abduction and ER – Refusal to move hip – Gait: unable to bear weight	– Preferred resting position of hip abduction and ER – ROM may be decreased – Pain severity ranges from mild to inability to bear weight – Gait: Ranges from decreased stance phase on affected side to non-weight-bearing	– Decreased hip IR, extension, abduction – Slight shortening of affected leg – Gait: Able to bear weight, more prominent lateral trunk sway over affected side than SA or ATS	– Preferred resting position: hip ER – Decreased hip IR, abduction
OTHER	*ORTHOPEDIC EMERGENCY	*MC cause of pediatric hip pain and limping		*MC hip disorder in preadolescents and adolescents

ATS, acute transient synovitis; ER, external rotation; IR, internal rotation; LCP, Legg-Calve-Perthes; MC, most common; ROM, range of motion; SA, septic arthritis; SCFE, slipped capital femoral epiphysis; URI, upper respiratory infection.

b. Most likely diagnosis: None of these diagnoses can be ruled out by history and exam alone. ATS, however, is the most common cause of pediatric acute painful hip, and is the most likely diagnosis for several additional reasons, including the patient's age, as SCFE tends to occur in adolescents while SA occurs largely in the first few years of life. The rapid onset of symptoms supports ATS or SA over LCP disease. A preceding upper respiratory infection (URI) can be associated with ATS. He also maintains the ability to bear weight, which is less likely in SA.

4. Acute hip pain in a child poses a diagnostic challenge. A septic joint is an orthopedic emergency and it is difficult to distinguish SA from ATS or other nonemergent causes of hip pain. Since ATS is a diagnosis of exclusion, further workup is necessary and the patient should be sent for urgent evaluation. You call ahead to the emergency and discuss your concerns as well as a recommended diagnostic workup, including a WBC, CRP, ESR, and a hip x-ray, with potential hip US and/or MRI.

5. After reviewing the bloodwork results and x-ray of the hips, you feel more reassured that the patient is less likely to have a septic hip, but recognizing that these tests do not exclude this diagnosis, you call back the physician who is completing the workup and you agree that a hip US is warranted. US is important for the detection of intracapsular effusions, and if present, an US-guided aspiration and culture can then be completed to rapidly test for septic effusion and may simultaneously offer immediate pain relief and improved hip movement by decreasing pressure within the joint space. Given the unremarkable bloodwork and radiographs, if culture of the hip effusion is also negative, you would discuss the diagnosis of ATS with the father. Management of ATS is conservative with relative rest. Nonsteroidal anti-inflammatory drugs (NSAIDs) can help relieve pain and may accelerate recovery. Resolution of more severe symptoms generally occurs in days, with lingering symptoms occurring for a week or two. Recovery may be accelerated by NSAIDs. If more severe symptoms persist for over a week or two after the initial presentation or if any residual hip symptoms persist for more than a month, it would be important to consider other pathologies.

6. As suggested in the title of the book by Cristian and Batmangelich, *Physical Medicine and Rehabilitation Patient-Centered Care: Mastering the Competencies*, patient-centered care for physiatrists revolves around the topic of systems-based practice, which includes delivering services and strategies to minimize costs while maintaining high-quality care. A thorough analysis of the risks and benefits for treatment planning is essential. Cristian and Batmangelich suggest the following as core competency guidelines to accomplish this goal:
   - *Identify relevant patient and situational characteristics pertinent to risk–benefit analysis.*
   - *Identify risks associated with a treatment or medical test and assign with value of high or low.*
   - *Identify benefits of test or treatment and assign with value of high or low.*
   - *Assign benefit value to test/treatment as high or low.*
   - *Review scientific literature, gather local expertise, and review applicable medical center rules, policies, procedures, or local laws for additional information.*
   - *Compare risks versus benefits and discuss these with patient, making note of the patient's wishes.*

7. It is certainly promising that the bloodwork and x-ray are normal. These do not, however, rule out the possibility of a septic hip. A septic joint is a serious acute condition that can cause permanent damage to the joint and permanent

disability to the child. As the symptoms only started 2 days ago, hip effusion or bony destruction may not yet be visible on x-ray. Additionally, he has a fever even while on ibuprofen, which may lead to underestimation of fever, a factor used in differentiating potential diagnoses. While you acknowledge and empathize with the father's frustration with waiting, you discuss that evaluation with the US not only allows visualization of a joint effusion that an x-ray may have missed but also allows for rapid US-guided aspiration and analysis of the joint fluid, which may help distinguish etiology and help guide treatment that could drastically alter the outcome for his son.

BIBLIOGRAPHY

Barr KP, Massagli TL. The use of milestones in physical medicine and rehabilitation residency education. In: Cristian A, Batmangelich S, eds. *Physical Medicine and Rehabilitation Patient-Centered Care: Mastering the Competencies.* Demos Medical Publishing; 2015:3–6.

Kang MS, Jeon JY, Park SS. Differential MRI findings of transient synovitis of the hip in children when septic arthritis is suspected according to symptom duration. *J Pediatr Orthop B.* 2020;29(3):297–303. https://doi.org/10.1097/BPB.0000000000000671

Murphy KP, Wunderlich CA. Orthopedics and musculoskeletal conditions. In: Alexander MA, Matthews DJ, eds. *Pediatric Rehabilitation: Principles and Practice.* 5th ed. Demos Medical Publishing; 2015:241–242. https://doi.org/10.1891/9781617052255.0010

Nouri A, Walmsley D, Pruszczynski B, et al. Transient synovitis of the hip: a comprehensive review. *J Pediatr Orthop B.* 2014;23(1):32–36. https://doi.org/10.1097/BPB.0b013e328363b5a3

Rossi R, Alexander M, Cuccurullo S. Pediatric rehabilitation. In: Cuccurullo S, ed. *Physical Medicine and Rehabilitation Board Review.* 2nd ed. Demos Medical Publishing; 2010:732–733.

Ryan DD. Differentiating transient synovitis of the hip from more urgent conditions. *Pediatr Ann.* 2016;45(6):e209–e213. https://doi.org/10.3928/00904481-20160427-01

Whitelaw CC, Varacallo M. Transient Synovitis. [Updated 2020 Jun 27]. In: *StatPearls [Internet].* StatPearls Publishing; January 2020. https://www.ncbi.nlm.nih.gov/books/NBK459181/. Jun 27, 2020. Accessed January 16, 2021.

12 Soft Tissue Impairments

R. Samuel Mayer

You are consulted on a 45-year-old woman with spastic diplegic cerebral palsy. She was recently admitted to a nursing facility as her elderly parents were no longer able to care for her. She ambulated with forearm crutches until 3 years ago. Her legs have become "so bent up" now that she can no longer stand.

Questions

1. What questions do you want to ask to learn more about her history? How will these questions help you understand her situation better?

2. What are particularly important components of her physical examination and why?

At the facility, they use a Hoyer lift to get her in and out of her wheelchair. She is in custodial care and gets no physical therapy (PT). Her aides do not perform range of motion stretches on her. She has no splints. She had serial casting as a child, which prevented surgery, but has had no such treatments since. She had botulinum toxin injections about 5 years ago by another provider, but they did not help. Currently, she takes baclofen 10 mg TID, and when she has increased the dose beyond that, it made her drowsy and confused. She does not think the baclofen helps.

On physical exam, she is alert and oriented and follows instructions well. Vitals are normal and body mass index (BMI) is 25. Upper limbs have normal strength, tone, and range of motion. In her lower limbs, strength is 5/5 within her range of motion. Tone is 4 on the modified Ashworth scale, but deep tendon reflexes are absent. Babinski is up-going bilaterally. She has 10-degree flexion contracture in her hips and 45-degree flexion contractures in her knees.

3. What is your differential diagnosis for the etiology of her functional decline?

4. What diagnostic tests would help sort through this differential diagnosis and help guide treatment?

X-rays of both her hips show mildly shallow acetabulum, while x-rays of knees and ankles are normal. Alkaline phosphatase is normal.

5. Outline your treatment plan.

The nursing facility does not provide PT at the custodial level of care, and the nursing home administrator refuses to pay for dynamic splints, which cost over $1,000.

6. How can you facilitate getting the patient the services she needs?

7. Please explain to the patient her diagnosis and treatment plan in lay terms.

Answers

1. Obtain information on her mobility and self-care. What help does she require, and what equipment does she use. What limits her mobility—stiffness, weakness, pain? What treatments has she had for this condition? What are her goals?

   This is important to develop a treatment plan that is patient-centered and maximizes her function.

2. On physical exam, you would want to assess cognition, strength, tone, and range of motion. You should look for evidence of spasticity as well as fixed contracture. This is important as treating spasticity without addressing contracture will be ineffective.

3. The primary diagnoses in the differential are spastic contracture, skeletal deformity (including overuse osteoarthritis), and heterotopic ossification.

4. X-rays would help rule out the latter two diagnoses. Alkaline phosphatase is often elevated before there are x-ray changes in heterotopic ossification.

5. If the patient desires to return to standing and walking, then treatment of the spastic contracture would be important. Treatment of spastic contracture requires treatment of both the spasticity and the contracture. Additional treatment of the spasticity might include phenol injections or an intrathecal baclofen pump. Treatment of the contracture requires prolonged stretch. This can be accomplished with serial casting or dynamic splints. Surgical lengthening of the hamstrings and iliopsoas can be considered.

6. This is a difficult problem for patients in custodial care. Facilities are not reimbursed for PT or durable medical equipment. If you have the skills, you can initiate serial casting, but must assure that the patient is seen frequently to watch for pressure sores. One way of appealing to the nursing facility to cover the dynamic splints is to convince them that the contractures can lead to bedsores, for which the facility can be cited by licensing agencies.

7. It is important to gauge her goals and what she is willing to do to correct this deformity. The contractures are the result of her muscles shortening due to continued tightening by the spasticity. Correcting this will require prolonged stretching, which can be painful. Another option may be to work more on wheelchair-level mobility and on gaining independence in transfers.

BIBLIOGRAPHY

Harvey LA, Katalinic OM, Herbert RD, et al. Stretch for the treatment and prevention of contracture: an abridged republication of a Cochrane Systematic Review. *J Physiother.* April 2017;63(2):67–75. Epub 2017 March 14. https://doi.org/10.1016/j.jphys.2017.02.014

Leung J, King C, Fereday S. Effectiveness of a programme comprising serial casting, botulinum toxin, splinting and motor training for contracture management: a randomized controlled trial. *Clin Rehabil.* June 2019;33(6):1035–1044. https://doi.org/10.1177/0269215519831337

A 28-year-old man with C7 tetraplegia returns to the clinic for the first time in 5 years. He has noted pressure sores developing on his buttocks recently.

Questions

1. What more do you want to know about the patient's history, comorbidities, and social situation? Please tell me why you are asking for these specifics.

2. How would you go about performing a physical exam on this patient? Why are these maneuvers/exam components important?

He lives alone in an accessible apartment. He has had the sores for about 3 months and is treating them himself with wet-to-dry dressing changes. He is in the wheelchair all day and performs weight shifts whenever he remembers. He uses a sliding board to transfer independently. He often voids in a diaper for bowel and bladder because transfers are difficult. He smokes one pack of cigarettes per day. He has two clean pressure injuries that do not have signs of infection located at his bilateral ischial tuberosities that are Stage III and about 7 cm in the largest diameter (Figure 12.1).

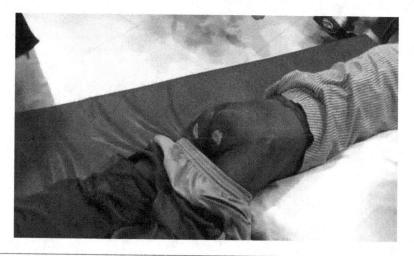

Figure 12.1 Stage III gluteal pressure sore.

3. What factors are contributing to his pressure sores?

4. What diagnostic test or tests would you order and why?

White blood cell count and c-reactive protein are normal.

5. Outline the treatment plan.

An insurance reviewer requests a peer-to-peer conversation regarding the durable medical equipment you recently prescribed, specifically the power wheelchair with tilt-in-space feature and custom cushion.

6. How do you justify the wheelchair?

7. In lay terms, explain to the patient his role in preventing recurrences of these sores.

Answers

1. You would need to know the constitutional information (weight gain, nutritional status), method of transfers, sitting time, weight shifts, bowel program, bladder program, and smoking history. Smoking increases the risk of pressure sores.

2. You would want to know the duration, location, stage, tunneling, signs of infection, and treatment.

3. Pressure sores develop because of lack of circulation due to unrelieved pressure on the area. Shear and moisture exacerbate this, as does tobacco use and malnutrition.

4. A complete blood count (CBC) and c-reactive protein or erythrocyte sedimentation rate would help rule out infection. If these are elevated, a bone scan might be considered. Pressure mapping may be helpful in prescribing a custom cushion.

5. He would need a referral to wound care, and need to be prone for much of the day. He should have an air mattress. Because he lives alone, a skilled nursing facility stay may be needed. He needs to be using intermittent catheterization or alternatively a Foley or suprapubic catheter, and should be on a daily bowel program. Smoking cessation and proper nutrition will help. Once he is sufficiently healed, a power tilt-in-space wheelchair with a cushion will help prevent recurrence.

6. This patient is at high risk of recurrence of pressure sores and might need extensive plastic surgery next time. This would result in prolonged hospitalization and skilled nursing facility admission. A power tilt-in-space chair will better enable him to independently relieve pressure. The cushion will also provide pressure relief.

7. Using motivational interviewing, engage the patient in a discussion of how willing and able he is to reduce his time upright, do pressure relief, stop smoking, and change his bowel and bladder program.

BIBLIOGRAPHY

Bergstrom N, Horn SD, Smout RJ, et al. The National Pressure Ulcer Long-Term Care Study: outcomes of pressure ulcer treatments in long-term care. *J Am Geriatr Soc.* 2005;53:1721. https://doi.org/10.1111/j.1532-5415.2005.53506.x

Chen Y, Devivo MJ, Jackson AB. Pressure ulcer prevalence in people with spinal cord injury: age-period-duration effects. *Arch Phys Med Rehabil.* 2005;86(6):1208–1213. https://doi.org/10.1016/j.apmr.2004.12.023

Groah SL, Schladen M, Pineda CG, et al. Prevention of pressure ulcers among people with spinal cord injury: a systematic review. *PM R.* 2015;7(6):613–636. https://doi.org/10.1016/j.pmrj.2014.11.014

A 28-year-old man with C7 AIS A tetraplegia returns to the clinic for the first time in 5 years. He is sent to you by his primary care physician who noted pressure sores on his physical exam.

Questions

1. What do you need to know from his history, review of systems (ROS), functional, and social history? Why is this important?

He has had them for about 3 months and is treating them himself with wet-to-dry dressing changes. He is in the wheelchair all day and performs weight shift whenever he remembers. He uses a sliding board to transfer independently. He often voids in a diaper for bowel and bladder because transfers are difficult. He has lost about 20 pounds over the last few months. He smokes one pack of cigarettes per day.

2. What are important elements of his exam?

He is afebrile. His BMI is 20. He has pressure sores on his buttocks. He has two clean pressure injuries that do not have signs of infection located at his bilateral ischial tuberosities that are Stage III and about 7 cm in the largest diameter. There is no surrounding erythema. There is no tunneling.

3. What factors are contributing to this patient's pressure sores?

4. What is the treatment plan for healing the pressure ulcers?

You decide with the patient that a tilt-in-space power wheelchair is needed to facilitate pressure relief. An insurance reviewer requests a peer-to-peer conversation regarding the durable medical equipment you recently prescribed, specifically the power wheelchair with tilt-in-space feature and cushion with pressure mapping.

5. How do you justify the wheelchair?

6. In lay terms, explain to him the importance of pressure relief.

Answers

1. You would want to know the length of time this has been going on and hw has he been treating this. You would need to know the constitutional information (weight gain, nutritional status), method of transfers, sitting time, weight shifts, bowel program, bladder program, and smoking history. Smoking increases the risk of pressure sores.

2. You should check his temperature (concerns for infection) and BMI (pressure from excess weight or, on the other hand, bony prominence from lack of adipose tissue). You would want to gauge the stage and size of the wounds, presence of tunneling, surrounding erythema, or purulent drainage.

3. Lack of pressure relief, poor sensation, shear from transfer, malnutrition, and smoking all contribute to his situation.

4. Treatment involves referral to the wound care team, home healthcare referral for the wound care, no more sitting upright until pressure ulcers heal, smoking cessation, and a bowel and bladder program in bed. There is weak evidence for the use of electrical stimulation or hyperbaric oxygen. Consideration should be given for a power tilt-in-space wheelchair to facilitate better pressure relief.

5. In lay terms, explain that moving pressure off the buttocks every 2 hours is essential. Explain how his limited sensation impacts this. Discuss smoking and malnutrition. Ask him what it would take for him to change his behaviors (motivational interviewing).

6. Power wheelchairs are very expensive, often costing as much as an automobile. Mobility in tetraplegia is challenging. Transfers to different elevations are difficult with his arm weakness. The patient requires a power wheelchair with adjustable heights to help with his transfers. Likewise, weight shift is not possible with his arm weakness, and given the history of pressure injury; he requires a tilt-in-space feature.

BIBLIOGRAPHY

Chen Y, Devivo MJ, Jackson AB. Pressure ulcer prevalence in people with spinal cord injury: age-period-duration effects. *Arch Phys Med Rehabil.* 2005;86(6):1208–1213. https://doi.org/10.1016/j.apmr.2004.12.023

Consortium for Spinal Cord Medicine Clinical Practice Guidelines. Pressure ulcer prevention and treatment following spinal cord injury: a clinical practice guideline for health-care professionals. *J Spinal Cord Med.* 2001;24 (suppl 1):S40–S101. https://doi.org/10.1080/10790268.2001.11753592

Groah SL, Schladen M, Pineda CG, et al. Prevention of pressure ulcers among people with spinal cord injury: a systematic review. *PM R.* 2015;7(6):613–636. https://doi.org/10.1016/j.pmrj.2014.11.014

Liu LQ, Moody J, Traynor M, et al. A systematic review of electrical stimulation for pressure ulcer prevention and treatment in people with spinal cord injuries. *J Spinal Cord Med.* 2014;37(6):703–718. https://doi.org/10.1179/20457 72314Y.0000000226

CASE 4

You are called to the burn unit to consult on a 50-year-old man with 50% burns from a house fire. He has just been extubated yesterday after a week on the ventilator and completed debridement surgery and initial skin grafting to all limbs and his trunk.

Questions

1. What are the key elements you need to know about his history and hospital course?

2. What are important components of physical exam and why?

He had fallen asleep while drinking and smoking, causing the fire. He has only been up to a chair once in his stay. Pain is managed with intravenous fentanyl patient-controlled anesthesia (PCA). He is alert and oriented. He is afebrile. He has orthostatic hypotension. His pulse ox on 3 L O^2 pnc is 91%. He has crackles in his bases. He has primarily third-degree burns on his neck, shoulders, chest, palms, and thighs. He has decreased sensation to light touch in the right lateral arm and dorsal hand. His left shoulder abduction and flexion are 0/5 strength, and his elbow, wrist, and finger extension are all 2/5 strength.

3. List his major impairments, the likely etiology of each, and how this will impact his rehabilitation.

4. What diagnostic tests would be helpful?

Electrodiagnostic studies are consistent with a posterior cord brachial plexopathy.

5. Outline a comprehensive rehabilitation program for this patient.

You are concerned that the patient's brachial plexopathy may have resulted from improper positioning in the ICU.

6. Describe steps in a quality improvement program that might address this issue.

At his outpatient follow-up visit, he comes with his wife. She reports that he has become very withdrawn. He refuses to leave the house. He was previously very social, but now he will not even let his friends come over.

7. How would you discuss issues of body image and depression with the patient and his wife?

Answers

1. You would want to know where the burns are and what complications has he had. Was there smoke inhalation injury? Does he have pain, and how is it managed? What further treatments or procedures are planned? What is his home situation like? Does he have family support? How is he functioning now? Does he use tobacco, alcohol, or illicit drugs?

2. It is important to have orthostatic vitals with a pulse oximetry. You should listen to his heart and lungs, as pulmonary complications are common. What surfaces are burned? The palms are important as this requires special splinting. A thorough neuro exam is important. These patients disproportionately develop peripheral neuropathy of critical illness as well as entrapment neuropathy.

3. He has the following impairments:

   Respiratory due to smoke inhalation, especially with prior tobacco abuse, as well as chest wall burns.

   Range of motion limitations to burns on shoulders and hands.

   Decreased sensation and strength in the right upper limb, likely due to brachial plexopathy.

4. Electrodiagnostic studies will be helpful to confirm a brachial plexopathy and aid with prognosis. There do not appear to be central nervous system (CNS) findings to warrant MRI at this time.

5. Positioning, gentle stretching, and splinting are important now. He will need dorsal splints for his hands due to palmar burns as well as his plexopathy. Early mobility reduces ICU length of stay and complications. Controlling his orthostasis with fluids and/or medications will be necessary to mobilize him. After grafts are sufficiently healed, compression garments can reduce cheloid formation. You would want psychology and substance abuse counseling involved in his care as well.

6. A retrospective chart review of the burn unit patients will be helpful to see if this is an isolated case or a pattern. Engage an interdisciplinary team with nursing, PT, occupational therapy, and the burn surgeons. It is important not to "finger-point" or blame and shame. Look at all the contributing factors, perhaps drawing a "fish-bone" chart with contributions from policies, environment, equipment, people, and patient factors. Once changes are made, examine outcomes and repeat the cycle.

7. You need to be sensitive in approaching this. Ask him what his concerns are. Ask about suicidal ideation and vegetative signs of depression. Check if he has relapsed into substance abuse. Explore his willingness to engage family

and friends for help. See if he is willing to see a psychologist; sometimes pastoral care can be an alternative.

BIBLIOGRAPHY

Dodd H, Fletchall S, Starnes C, et al. Current concepts burn rehabilitation, Part II: long-term recovery. *Clin Plast Surg.* 2017;44(4):713–728. https://doi.org/10.1016/j.cps.2017.05.013

Jacobson K, Fletchall S, Dodd H, et al. Current concepts burn rehabilitation, Part I: care during hospitalization. *Clin Plast Surg.* 2017;44(4):703–712. https://doi.org/10.1016/j.cps.2017.05.003

Kornhaber R, Wilson A, Abu-Qamar MZ, et al. Adult burn survivors' personal experiences of rehabilitation: an integrative review. *Burns.* 2014;40(1):17–29. https://doi.org/10.1016/j.burns.2013.08.003

Strong AL, Agarwal S, Cederna PS, et al. Peripheral neuropathy and nerve compression syndromes in burns. *Clin Plast Surg.* 2017;44(4):793–803. https://doi.org/10.1016/j.cps.2017.05.010

13 Spinal Impairments

Bryt A. Christensen

A 51-year-old male presents to your outpatient clinic complaining of severe back pain and difficulty walking.

Questions

1. What more do you want to know about the patient's history, comorbidities, and social situation? Please tell me why you are asking for these specifics.

2. How would you go about performing a physical exam on this patient? Why are these maneuvers/exam components important?

The patient has had back pain on and off for many years. He has tried physical therapy in the past. His pain has been shooting down his legs for a few weeks, and yesterday he started having trouble walking. He also complains that he lost control of his bowels before he came to the office, and he feels like his bum is numb. His strength testing is difficult due to pain, he has decreased light touch and pinprick sensation in the legs, his reflexes are brisk, and he has an upgoing toe response to the Babinski test. His rectal tone is absent.

3. What is the differential diagnosis for this patient? Tell me the most likely diagnosis and why.

4. What diagnostic test or tests would you order and why?

Upon review of the hospital record, you see that the patient received a STAT thoracic and lumbar MRI that showed a large disc extrusion at the T12-L1 level causing impingement of the conus of the spinal cord.

5. Outline the treatment plan. Please tell me the initial treatment and next steps if that fails.

After you finish seeing patients that day in clinic, you find out that the gentleman you had emergency transferred for cauda equina syndrome earlier had called in the day before but was unable to see you because your clinic was full. The receptionist made his appointment for today instead.

6. How might your clinic better triage patients when they call asking to be seen?

Before the patient was transferred by ambulance to the hospital he expressed concern about going to the hospital. He stated that he had a sister pass away there recently. He said he rather not go.

7. How might you explain the urgency of the situation to this patient and reassure him of the care he will receive at the hospital?

Answers

1. What is the location of pain (any radiating symptoms [i.e., into the thighs/ legs]), intensity of pain, aggravating/alleviating factors, history of trauma or back surgery, any associated weakness, any associated bladder or bowel incontinence, any fevers, and any history of cancer and associated numbness or tingling in a saddle pelvic distribution? These questions help identify if there is a need for an urgent workup and/or possible urgent surgical referral needs (i.e., loss of bowel or bladder control, saddle anesthesia, severe or progressive weakness) or potential infection. All other symptoms can be worked up in a standard outpatient fashion. Location and aggravating/alleviating factors and history help with the development of a differential diagnosis.

2. The physical exam should at least include a detailed lower extremity neurologic exam (strength, sensation, reflexes, primitive reflexes) and musculoskeletal exam (inspection, palpation, range of motion of the low back and sacroiliac [SI] joints, provocative tests, and gait analysis). If bowel and bladder control is an issue, then an exam for rectal tone is necessary to know if emergency surgery is needed for cauda equina syndrome.

3. Cauda equina syndrome is the most likely diagnosis given the loss of strength, loss of sensation, loss of bowel control, weakness, and brisk reflexes. The exact cause of the syndrome could be a disc herniation, severe central stenosis in the thoracic or thoracolumbar junction, a tumor, or an infection (i.e., an epidural abscess). The brisk reflexes and upgoing toes on a Babinski test suggest an upper motor neuron issue so the lesion must be at the conus of the cord or higher.

4. Given that this patient is in an outpatient setting, he should be immediately transferred via ambulance to the ED of a hospital capable of emergency spinal surgery. The hospital should be advised of his coming, along with the likely diagnosis and the recommendation that a STAT thoracic and lumbar MRI with and without contrast should not be delayed. The on-call neurosurgeon or spine surgeon should be notified and apprised of the patient's situation and transfer. No outpatient test is appropriate at this time.

5. The treatment of a large disc extrusion causing severe neurological symptoms and especially when causing cauda equina syndrome is immediate surgical decompression to relieve pressure off the affected spinal cord region.

6. Some conditions are much more urgent than others. The receptionists should be educated and policy should be in place to ask for certain "red flag" symptoms patients may be having when they call in for an appointment. If certain "red flag" symptoms are present, patients could be triaged to the appropriate care setting per the policy in place. This would help patients like the one in this scenario receive the care they need in the most timely manner.

7. "Sir, you may have a very serious condition in your spine that needs to be taken care of immediately. If we do not get you the appropriate care right away then the pain and weakness that you have could become permanent. Our hospital has excellent doctors and staff, and I know you will be in good hands. I will personally call ahead to let them know you are coming, and I will be in touch with you to check on how you are doing throughout your stay."

BIBLIOGRAPHY

Crocker M, Fraser G, Boyd E, et al. The value of interhospital transfer and emergency MRI for suspected cauda equina syndrome: a 2-year retrospective study. *Ann R Coll Surg Engl.* September 2008;90(6):513–516. https://doi.org/10.1308/003588408X301154

Goodman BP. Disorders of the cauda equina. *Continuum (Minneap Minn).* April 2018;24(2, Spinal Cord Disorders):584–602. https://doi.org/10.1212/CON.0000000000000584

Hoeritzauer I, Pronin S, Carson A, et al. The clinical features and outcome of scan-negative and scan-positive cases in suspected cauda equina syndrome: a retrospective study of 276 patients. *J Neurol.* 2018;265(12):2916–2926. https://doi.org/10.1007/s00415-018-9078-2

CASE 2

A 36-year-old woman presents to your outpatient office complaining of low back pain that she has had for 7 years, following the birth of her third child. She is finding it more difficult to sit for extended periods of time, especially on the bleachers at her oldest son's basketball games recently.

Questions

1. What more do you want to know about the patient's history, comorbidities, and social situation? Please tell me why you are asking for these specifics.

2. How would you go about performing a physical exam on this patient? Why are these maneuvers/exam components important?

She has no "red flags" and no radicular pain. Her average pain is a 6/10. Sitting worsens her pain while lying down or standing up alleviates it some. She has no kyphoscoliosis and a full range of motion. Straight leg raising is negative. No pain is reported with extension or lateral bending. She has point tenderness over the bilateral SI joints, positive FABER (flexion, abduction, external rotation; for buttocks but not groin pain), positive compression and distraction of the SI joints, and bilateral positive Gaenslen's tests.

3. What is the differential diagnosis for this patient? Tell me the most likely diagnosis and why.

4. What diagnostic test or tests would you order and why?

X-ray of the SI joint shows no visible pathology. Human leukocyte antigen B27 (HLA-B27) and erythrocyte sedimentation rate (ESR) labs are normal.

5. Outline the treatment plan. Please tell me the initial treatment and next steps if that fails.

The patient fails conservative treatment and comes back to your office 4 weeks later in worsening pain. She is no longer able to sit for any length of time for her job and is fearful of losing her job because of it. She would like to have an injection performed immediately for relief of pain; however, her insurance requires prior authorization.

6. How might you address this patient and explain why prior authorization is needed before doing a procedure? What factors would you incorporate in addressing this situation?

You perform an SI joint injection for her. Three days later, you learn that the triamcinolone you injected has been recalled by the pharmaceutical company because it may have been contaminated with *Staphylococcus* from a faulty seal.

7. Tell me in lay terms how you would explain this to the patient.

Answers

1. When a patient presents with back pain, it is important to ask about "red flags" symptoms and signs: fevers, history of cancer, progressive weakness, and bowel or bladder incontinence. Red flag symptoms and signs would alert to a more serious cause of the pain requiring more aggressive and timely diagnosis and treatment. Next, further define the character and severity of the pain and ask about aggravating and alleviating factors. It is also important to ask what the impact of the pain on her function so appropriate treatment is initiated.

2. First. inspect the spine. Look for spinal deformity. Palpate over the spinous processes, paraspinals, SI joint, trochanteric and ischial bursae. Test spinal range of motion. A lower extremity neurological exam checking for sensation, reflexes, and strength should be performed to rule out any neurological compromise. Specific tests for common etiologies of back pain should be performed:

   Radicular pain: Straight leg raising, femoral stretch, neurologic exam.

   Facet cause: Facet loading, tenderness with palpation of the lumbar paraspinal area.

   SI joint pain: Tenderness to palpation of SI joint and provocative testing: Gaenslen (Figure 13.1), FABER/Patrick's test, ASIS distraction (supine), sacral compression (side lying).

3. SI joint pain, discogenic low back pain, mechanical low back pain. There are many causes to low back pain, but given the results of this patient's physical exam (negative tests for radicular and facet causes and positive tests for SI joint pain) bilateral SI joint pain is the most likely cause for this patient.

4. An x-ray of the pelvis is indicated (anteroposterior angled and bilateral oblique views of the SI joints) to look for a cause to the SI joint pain. An MRI is not warranted at this point as the patient has no neurological signs or symptoms and no "red flags." Lab work should include HLA-B27 and an ESR to exclude inflammatory sacroiliitis.

5. Initial treatment would include rehabilitative therapy, including manual therapy, and modalities (ultrasound, iontophoresis, electrical stimulation), stretching (specifically of the hamstrings), strengthening of the legs and gluteus muscle groups, and core strengthening. An anti-inflammatory medication, if not contraindicated, should be used for a short duration. If conservative management is not helping or is not tolerated, an SI joint corticosteroid injection may be helpful. Furthermore, prolotherapy and platelet-rich plasma therapy have shown promising evidence for their use. Performing lateral branch radiofrequency ablation might also be considered. Fusion of the SI joint is a last-resort procedure. Risks of procedures should be well described

to the patient such as infection, bleeding, worsening of pain or lack of effect, and so on.

6. It is important to understand the insurance process for your patients as the insurers often dictates what treatment is covered and when it is considered appropriate. Explain that some insurers require that the physician submit proof of medical necessity, via the patient medical record, to have a procedure authorized. Until prior authorization is obtained, any cost of treatment given could be the responsibility of the patient. It could be explained that the patient could pay for the procedure upfront and then obtain payment for the procedure from their insurer, but they would be at risk that the procedure is not authorized. You should be familiar with how insurers handle these situations or have someone within your office who handles these kinds of questions so you can focus on patient care.

7. "We were informed by the company who makes the medication that we injected into your SI joint that it could have been contaminated and could cause an infection. You may or may not have a reaction to it. I am happy to discuss what to look out for and what to do if there is a problem. We will do some blood tests now to see if you have an infection. You should look out for any redness or hot spots at the injection site. Watch for any increase in pain at the injection site, or if you develop new neck pain. Take your temperature daily for the next several days, and let me know immediately if you have a fever."

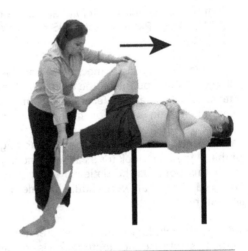

Figure 13.1 Gaenslen's maneuver.

BIBLIOGRAPHY

Cohen SP, Chen Y, Neufeld NJ. Sacroiliac joint pain: a comprehensive review of epidemiology, diagnosis and treatment. *Expert Rev Neurother.* January 2013;13(1):99–116. https://doi.org/10.1586/ern.12.148

Hoffman MD, Agnish V. Functional outcome from sacroiliac joint prolotherapy in patients with sacroiliac joint instability. *Complement Ther Med.* April 2018;37:64–68. https://doi.org/10.1016/j.ctim.2018.01.014

Quijano DAS, Loperena EO. Sacroiliac joint interventions. *Phys Med Rehabil Clin N Am.* February 2018;29(1):171–183. https://doi.org/10.1016/j.pmr.2017.09.004

An 11-year-old female presents to your office with her mother. The mother states that the patient was undergoing a routine physical examination by her family doctor for sports participation when she was found to have scoliosis. She was then referred to you for management.

Questions

1. What more do you want to know about the patient's history, comorbidities, and social situation? Please tell me why you are asking for these specifics.

2. How would you go about performing a physical exam on this patient? Why are these maneuvers/exam components important?

She does not complain of any neurologic symptoms, has a normal birth history, childhood, and normal growth. There is no family history of scoliosis of any kind. On exam you find no dysmorphic anatomy and no signs of congenital disease. She is neurologically intact with normal strength, sensation, and reflexes. Her spine has a rightward thoracolumbar curve with the left shoulder sitting lower, and there is protrusion of the right rib cage and scapula.

3. What is the differential diagnosis for this patient? Tell me the most likely diagnosis and why.

4. What diagnostic test or tests would you order and why?

The spine radiographs show a 20-degree curvature of the thoracic spine with a 15-degree compensatory lumbar curve. Pelvic radiographs show a Risser grade of 3.

5. Outline the treatment plan. Please tell me the initial treatment and next steps if that fails.

The patient expresses concern about her appearance, how she already has a hard time fitting in at school with the popular girls, and how now she must also deal with a deformed body.

6. How might you provide care in this situation?

The patient's mother expresses confusion over the diagnosis and treatment plan when she asks, "so my daughter was born with a deformed back and needs to have surgery?"

7. Explain in lay terms what the diagnosis and treatment plan is.

Answers

1. Pertinent questions to ask regarding this patient's history should include the patient's birth history and pediatric milestones obtainment history. You should also ask about growth and puberty. Other important questions would include family history of congenital, neuromuscular, or idiopathic causes of scoliosis. If there is an abnormal birth history, known congenital disorders, or delay in milestone achievement then there may be a congenital or neuromuscular cause to the scoliosis. Family history of any such disorders would also help tip you off toward a congenital, neuromuscular, or idiopathic cause to the scoliosis. Other important questions to ask would include questions regarding any neurological symptoms (numbness, tingling, burning, weakness, etc.). These questions will help you understand the severity and will help decide management.

2. Key components of the physical exam include inspection/observation. It would be important to look for any dysmorphic features and skin abnormalities, such as café-au-lait spots, dimpling of skin or tuft of hair over low back, long fingers, or chest deformities. Finding these features may lead to a diagnosis of a neurogenic disorder and help determine the underlying cause of the scoliosis. A thorough neurologic exam of the cranial nerves and extremities (sensation, reflexes, and strength) should be performed to determine if there is any central nervous system involvement and/or if there is any signs of nerve impairment or damage. A musculoskeletal exam (inspection/palpation of spine and limbs, range of motion of spine, chest expansion, gait analysis) should be performed to determine if the scoliosis or underlying cause is affecting function. The exam will help determine what further studies to order and what treatment and consults may be in order.

3. Adolescent idiopathic scoliosis, congenital scoliosis, and neuromuscular scoliosis. Adolescent idiopathic scoliosis is the likely diagnosis given that there is no other history or features and signs on exam that would point to a congenital or neuromuscular cause.

4. Appropriate diagnostic tests would include standing upright, plain radiographs of the spine (cervical, thoracic, and lumbar to measure degree of scoliosis), as well as a pelvic radiograph (to measure Risser grade and better predict bone growth potential).

5. If the curvature is less than 40 degrees, management is usually conservative and could include bracing, with repeat x-rays in 6 months to a year. Bracing requires that the patient where the brace approximately 23 hours per day and could include a Milwaukee brace, Boston brace, or the Charleston brace. If the curve progresses beyond 40 degrees or causes neurological or respiratory compromise, a surgical consult should be obtained.

6. Peer counseling can be beneficial if there is a support group in your area or online with other patients like her. Also, given the patient's response it would be appropriate to provide a referral for psychological counseling to help her manage her concerns and feelings.

7. (An explanation in lay terms may go something like this.) Ma'am, your daughter, most likely, has developed a curve in her spine as she has started to grow. That curve may continue to worsen until she stops growing. We can provide bracing for her that can potentially stop the curve from getting any worse. She may need to wear a brace until she stops growing. We will obtain x-rays of her spine periodically to look for any changes. If the curve gets too severe then we may need to have her see a surgeon that could straighten it with surgery.

BIBLIOGRAPHY

Choudhry MN, Ahmad Z, Verma R. Adolescent idiopathic scoliosis. *Open Orthop J.* 2016;10:143–154. https://doi.org/10.2174/1874325001610010143

El-Hawary R, Chukwunyerenwa C. Update on evaluation and treatment of scoliosis. *Pediatr Clin North Am.* 2014;61(6):1223–1241. https://doi.org/10.1016/j.pcl.2014.08.007

Horne JP, Flannery R, Usman S. Adolescent idiopathic scoliosis: diagnosis and management. *Am Fam Physician.* 2014;89(3):193–198.

CASE 4

A 48-year-old, right-handed man was referred to your clinic by his primary care provider. He complains of neck and right-hand pain.

Questions

1. What more do you want to know about the patient's history, comorbidities, and social situation? Please tell me why you are asking for these specifics.

2. How would you go about performing a physical exam on this patient? Why are these maneuvers/exam components important?

His symptoms are off and on but much worse when suddenly, at work, he felt a sharp, shooting pain down his arm. Pain is in the lateral half of his hand and fingers and up his lateral forearm. He is having a hard time gripping and lifting. No gait, bladder, or bowel changes. No fevers, recent weight loss, or history of cancer. He has decreased sensation in the C6 and C7 distribution, and 4/5 strength of the finger abductors and wrist extensors, his brachioradialis deep tendon reflex is absent on the right, the Hoffman's test is negative, and right-sided Spurling's maneuver causes shooting pain from the neck into the arm.

3. What is the differential diagnosis for this patient? Tell me the most likely diagnosis and why.

4. What diagnostic test or tests would you order and why?

Cervical x-rays show multilevel degenerative changes and narrowing of the disc space at C5 to C6 and C6 to C7, without any instability. Cervical MRI shows a C5 to C6 and a C6 to C7 posterior lateral disc bulge with right-sided neural foraminal narrowing (Figure 13.2). Nerve conduction study (NCS)/electromyography (EMG), if ordered, reveals a C6 and C7 radiculopathies.

5. Outline the treatment plan. Please tell me the initial treatment and next steps if that fails.

The patient works as a mechanic. He asks for release from work due to his condition.

6. Is a work release appropriate for this patient? Would you give a full or a partial release and for how long?

He is now very worried that he is going to have to have surgery. "I don't want a fusion like my brother," he states.

7. Tell me in lay terms how you would react to his worry and comment?

Answers

1. When were the onset of symptoms (gradual versus. sudden), exact location of pain, aggravating/alleviating factors, is there any numbness or tingling, any associated weakness, history of trauma, any history of neck or arm surgery, any associated bladder or bowel dysfunction, any fevers, and any history of cancer. Each of these questions help to determine the importance of quick intervention versus being able to try conservative treatments. These questions also help distinguish between multiple potential causes of the chief complaint.

2. A detailed neurological exam of the extremities is important. Test for sensation of the extremities, manual muscle testing, deep tendon reflexes, Hoffman's test, Babinski test, Spurling's maneuver, Phalen's maneuver, Tinel's test at the wrist, cervical range of motion, and inspection and palpation of the cervical spine.

3. Cervical radiculopathy, cervical stenosis, brachial plexopathy, peripheral neuropathy (including entrapment neuropathies), and forearm tendinopathy. His symptoms and physical exam is typical of a cervical radiculopathy given the weakness, sensation loss, reflexes, and associated neck pain.

4. A cervical MRI without contrast would be the diagnostic test of choice to look for causes of a cervical radiculopathy and should be ordered without delay due to the associated weakness found on exam. Cervical spine x-rays are also appropriate with flexion and extension views to rule out any instability. An EMG would also be appropriate to look for a corresponding cause in relation to the MRI findings and to further characterize the acuity of the radiculopathy.

5. Ice/heat and massage are used for symptom management. Nonsteroidal anti-inflammatory drugs (NSAIDs; if no medical contraindications) can be prescribed. An oral steroid taper (e.g., Medrol Dose Pak) can be helpful to minimize inflammation and reduce pain while the patient is undergoing workup or conservative treatment. Neuropathic medications (such as gabapentin, pregabalin, tricyclic antidepressants, duloxetine) can help to treat the neuropathic component of pain. Opioids could be considered only for short-term use and only for severe pain and loss of function. Physical therapy can often help resolve radicular pain and is typically considered the first-line treatment (manual treatment, modalities, traction, range of motion exercises). Cervical epidural steroid injections can decrease pain and may be indicated in this case if an identifiable cause of cervical radicular pain is found. Surgical referral would be appropriate and indicated if the patient does not respond to conservative treatment and has ongoing or worsening weakness.

6. A full work release is very reasonable and warranted in this situation. Two weeks for rest, therapy, and obtaining ordered tests with a follow-up visit to reevaluate and go over test results would be reasonable. He could do more harm working as a mechanic.

7. Many people with your condition do not end up needing surgery. With treatment we may be able to get you relief from your pain and the weakness may improve. We do need to be careful with the weakness you have, though. Surgery may be able to help those nerves recover, if needed. We will go over your test results next time and see how you are improving.

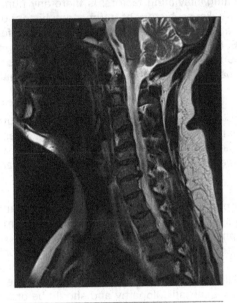

Figure 13.2 Cervical spine MRI revealing a C6 to C7 posterior lateral disc bulge.

BIBLIOGRAPHY

Childress MA, Becker BA. Nonoperative management of cervical radiculopathy. *Am Fam Physician*. May 1, 2016;93(9):746–754.
Woods BI, Hilibrand AS. Cervical radiculopathy: epidemiology, etiology, diagnosis, and treatment. *J Spinal Disord Tech*. June 2015;28(5):E251–E259. https://doi.org/10.1097/BSD.0000000000000284

CASE 5

A 49-year-old, left-handed female presents to your clinic with low back pain. She states that she has had the pain for years and it has gradually gotten much worse. In the past, it would come and go and now it is more persistent on a daily basis, especially in the morning and when she stays in any position for too long.

Questions

1. What more do you want to know about the patient's history, comorbidities, and social situation? Please tell me why you are asking for these specifics.

2. How would you go about performing a physical exam on this patient? Why are these maneuvers/exam components important?

Her pain is in the low back with no weakness or numbness. She does not have any history of trauma, surgery, or cancer. She does not have any bowel or bladder incontinence nor fevers. Her strength, sensation, reflexes, and gait are all within normal limitations. A Babinski test reveals down going of the toes bilaterally. She has a mild degree of lumbar scoliosis, mild pain to palpation of the lumbar paravertebral muscles, and worsening pain with extension maneuvers of the lumbar spine. FABER test is negative and there is no pain over the SI joints.

3. What is the differential diagnosis for this patient? Tell me the most likely diagnosis and why.

4. What diagnostic test or tests would you order and why?

Lumbar posteroanterior (PA) and lateral x-rays reveal lumbosacral spondylosis with moderate to severe facet joint arthropathy.

5. Outline the treatment plan. Please tell me initial treatment and next steps if that fails.

She returns to clinic after attending only one physical therapy session. She states that she cannot afford the co-pay on her insurance. She is, however, highly motivated to get better. Her insurance requires conservative treatment prior to any procedures.

6. What options might she have?

The patient returns after 4 weeks of performing her home exercise regimen you prescribed and still has no change in her pain and function. She asks, "What is radiofrequency ablation?"

7. Explain radiofrequency ablation in lay terms.

Answers

1. What is the exact location of pain (any radiating symptoms [i.e., into the thighs/legs]), intensity of pain, aggravating/alleviating factors, history of trauma or back surgery, any associated weakness, any associated bladder or bowel incontinence, any fevers, and any history of cancer and associated numbness or tingling in a saddle pelvic distribution? These questions help identify if there is a need for an urgent workup and/or possible urgent surgical referral needs (i.e., loss of bowel or bladder control, saddle anesthesia, severe or progressive weakness) or potential infection. All other symptoms can be worked up in a standard outpatient fashion. Location and aggravating/alleviating factors and history help with development of a differential diagnosis.

2. The most pertinent exam elements would include sensation of lower limbs, manual muscle testing, deep tendon reflexes, Babinski test, inspection and palpation of the lumbar spine and sacrum, range of motion of the lumbar spine, straight leg raising, facet joint loading, and special SI joint tests. If bowel and bladder control is an issue, then an exam for rectal tone is necessary to know if emergency surgery is needed.

3. Differential diagnosis includes lumbar facet arthropathy, degenerative intervertebral disc disease or an annular tear, lumbar myofascial pain, vertebral compression fracture, lumbar spondylolisthesis/spondylolysis, and SI joint arthropathy. Given her history and physical exam, lumbar facet arthropathy is the most likely diagnosis.

4. Diagnostic studies could include lumbar x-rays, lumbar CT (only if an MRI is contraindicated), or lumbar MRI without contrast. It would be appropriate to attempt a course of conservative measures prior to obtaining imaging. A lumbar x-ray would be the most appropriate radiographic study (at least PA and lateral views; oblique views would aid in diagnosis of facet arthropathy and flexion/extension view with listhesis). An MRI should be reserved for patients with neurologic deficits or symptoms, or for those with a high certainty of fracture, infection, cancer, or failure of conservative treatment.

5. Conservative measures such as ice, heat, massage, acupuncture, chiropractic/osteopathic manipulation, and/or physical therapy (manual treatment, modalities, core strengthening, and range of motion exercises) are first-line treatments. NSAIDs can relieve pain but should be used on a short basis if no contraindications (history of gastroesophageal reflux disease [GERD], cardiovascular disease, or decreased kidney function). Opioids should be used short term only for severe pain and loss of function. Facet joint corticosteroid injections or medial branch blocks with resultant radiofrequency ablation can be used if conservative management fails.

6. You could prescribe a home therapy program that she could follow. Other exercise routines such as yoga or Pilates can be performed at home with instructional videos readily available. She should be counseled about safety in doing these routines.

7. Radiofrequency ablation is an outpatient procedure done using small needles to cauterize or burn the nerves that carry the pain signal from your painful lumbar joints to your brain. By cauterizing the nerves, it causes them to die back, for a time, therefore relieving pain from the joint.

BIBLIOGRAPHY

Manchikanti L, Hirsch JA, Falco FJ, et al. Management of lumbar zygapophysial (facet) joint pain. *World J Orthop.* May 18, 2016;7(5):315–337. https://doi.org/10.5312/wjo.v7.i5.315

Perolat R, Kastler A, Nicot B, et al. Facet joint syndrome: from diagnosis to interventional management. *Insights Imaging.* October 2018;9(5):773–789. https://doi.org/10.1007/s13244-018-0638-x

A 74-year-old female comes to your office with a chief complaint of back pain for 3 weeks that has progressively gotten worse since the onset.

Questions

1. What more do you want to know about the patient's history, comorbidities, and social situation? Please tell me why you are asking for these specifics.

2. How would you go about performing a physical exam on this patient? Why are these maneuvers/exam components important?

Her pain is located over the mid- to lower back (thoracolumbar) area. She denies any weakness and pain or numbness going down the thighs or legs. Her pain ranges from a persistent 6 to 10/10. Pain tends to get worse when bending forward. She does recall falling a few weeks back when rolling out of bed. She does not have any history of surgery or cancer. She does not have any bowel or bladder incontinence and does not report any fever. Her strength, sensation, reflexes, and gait are all within normal limitations. A Babinski test reveals down-going toes bilaterally. She has a mild degree of lumbar scoliosis and severe pain to palpation of the midline thoracolumbar junction.

3. What is the differential diagnosis for this patient? Tell me the most likely diagnosis and why.

4. What diagnostic test or tests would you order and why?

An MRI confirms your suspicion of a superior endplate vertebral compression fracture at L1. There is no retropulsion of bone, but there is a vertebral height loss of 25%. There is bone marrow edema seen on T2 images, indicating an acute–subacute fracture.

5. Outline the treatment plan. Please tell me the initial treatment and next steps if that fails.

The patient fails conservative treatment with pain medication and a brace. She lives alone and only has a neighbor that can help her some.

6. How care might be facilitated?

She expresses some confusion over why she may have "cement" placed in her back.

7. How might the situation be explained in lay terms to help her understand?

Answers

1. What is the location of pain (any radiating symptoms [i.e., into the thighs/legs]), intensity of pain, aggravating/alleviating factors, history of trauma or back surgery, any associated weakness, any associated bladder or bowel incontinence, any fevers, and any history of cancer and associated numbness or tingling in a saddle pelvic distribution? These questions help identify if there is a need for an urgent workup and/or possible urgent surgical referral needs (i.e., loss of bowel or bladder control, saddle anesthesia, severe or progressive weakness) or potential infection. All other symptoms can be worked up in a standard outpatient fashion. Location and aggravating/alleviating factors and history help with the development of a differential diagnosis.

2. The most pertinent exam elements would include sensation of lower limbs, manual muscle testing, deep tendon reflexes, Babinski test, inspection and palpation of the lumbar spine and sacrum, range of motion of the lumbar spine, straight leg raising, facet joint loading, and special SI joint tests. If bowel and bladder control is an issue, then an exam for rectal tone is necessary to know if emergency surgery is needed.

3. The differential diagnosis could include vertebral compression fracture, discitis/osteomyelitis, spinal tumor, thoracolumbar spondylolysis/spondylolisthesis, facet syndrome, and myalgia. A vertebral compression fracture is most likely, given the patient's age, history of a fall and then onset of pain, and with pain of palpation of the midline spine.

4. The next best step would be to obtain an MRI of the thoracic and lumbar spines. An MRI would be the diagnostic modality of choice to not only evaluate a potential vertebral compression fracture but would also help define the age of the fracture and give important details for interventional decision-making. An MRI would also help to evaluate for potential tumors (spinal metastasis) or an infection. If an MRI is contraindicated, a CT scan would be appropriate.

5. Treatment would include pain control, and NSAIDs should be avoided to not delay bone healing. Restrictions of weight-bearing activity (walking aids if indicated), and potential fracture stabilization (bracing, vertebral augmentation such as vertebroplasty/kyphoplasty, or surgical treatment). Fracture stabilization is important to prevent the worsening of the fracture while it is healing. At minimum, a lumbar brace (lumbosacral orthosis [LSO]) should be ordered. A cruciform-anterior-spinal-hyperextension orthosis (CASH) brace helps place the lumbar spine in extension and prevents the potential damaging forces of flexion on a compression fracture and would be indicated (Figure 13.3). Indications for vertebral augmentation include failure of pain control despite conservative treatment/bracing, worsening of fracture despite conservative treatment, minimal to no retropulsion of fracture, and no neurologic deficit due to the fracture. Surgery is indicated if there is neurological compromise

often caused by retropulsion of the fracture with failure of conservative treatment. There should also be a plan for osteoporosis testing and treatment.

6. The patient needs vertebral augmentation, which has been shown to reduce mortality from osteoporotic compression fractures with associated reduction of pain and increase in function. She will need a referral to a physician who performs this procedure and will need home health set up to help her with her home recovery.

7. Your fall caused one of your spinal bones to squish down and break. It is not healing well. We can have some cement placed in the bone to act as an internal cast to help relief your pain.

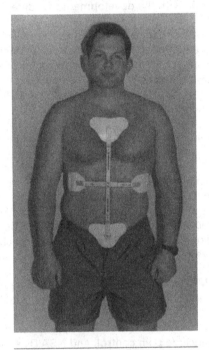

Figure 13.3 A cruciform-anterior-spinal-hyperextension orthosis.

BIBLIOGRAPHY

Beall D, Lorio MP, Yun BM, et al. Review of vertebral augmentation: an updated meta-analysis of the effectiveness. *Int J Spine Surg*. June 2018;12(3):295–321. https://doi.org/10.14444/5036

Hirsch JA, Chandra RV, Carter NS, et al. Number needed to treat with vertebral augmentation to save a life. *Am J Neuroradiol*. January 2020;41(1):178–182. https://doi.org/10.3174/ajnr.A6367

Wong C, McGirt M. Vertebral compression fractures: a review of current management and multimodal therapy. *J Multidiscip Healthc*. 2013;6:205–221. https://doi.org/10.2147/JMDH.S31659

A 29-year-old male comes to your clinic because of 3 days of low back pain. He was referred to your clinic from the ED, where he went yesterday when his pain suddenly got much worse.

Questions

1. What more do you want to know about the patient's history, comorbidities, and social situation? Please tell me why you are asking for these specifics.

2. How would you go about performing a physical exam on this patient? Why are these maneuvers/exam components important?

He has a normal exam except for some tenderness in the bilateral lumbar paraspinal muscles and decreased range of motion of the lumbar spine due to pain.

3. What is the differential diagnosis for this patient? Tell me the most likely diagnosis and why.

4. What diagnostic test or tests would you order and why?

His lumbar spine AP and lateral x-rays show no abnormalities.

5. Outline the treatment plan. Please tell me the initial treatment and next steps if that fails.

Ordering inappropriate or unnecessary tests increases healthcare costs, utilizes important healthcare resources, and may expose patients to unnecessary risks. It is easy to feel the need to order tests during a patient's first encounter

6. Describe how you might initiate a quality improvement project in your practice to reduce the number of unnecessary radiographs, CT scans, and MRIs ordered for acute back pain.

The patient wants something stronger than NSAIDs and acetaminophen for his pain. He is demanding "real" pain medicine. He says the other medication is not going to work, and he cannot stand the pain anymore.

7. How would you respond to this patient?

Answers

1. What is the location of pain (any radiating symptoms [i.e., into the thighs/legs]), intensity of pain, aggravating/alleviating factors, history of trauma or back surgery, any associated weakness, any associated bladder or bowel incontinence, any fevers, and any history of cancer and associated numbness or tingling in a saddle pelvic distribution? These questions help identify if there is a need for an urgent workup and/or possible urgent surgical referral needs (i.e., loss of bowel or bladder control, saddle anesthesia, severe or progressive weakness) or potential infection. All other symptoms can be worked up in a standard outpatient fashion. Location and aggravating/alleviating factors and history help with the development of a differential diagnosis.

2. The physical exam should at least include a lower extremity neurologic exam (strength, sensation, reflexes, primitive reflexes) and musculoskeletal exam (inspection, palpation, range of motion of the low back and SI joints, provocative tests, gait analysis).

3. Differential diagnosis includes mechanical low back pain, lumbar facet arthropathy, degenerative intervertebral disc disease or an annular tear, vertebral compression fracture, lumbar spondylolisthesis/spondylolysis, and SI joint arthropathy. Given the history and physical exam, mechanical low back pain is the most likely diagnosis, but imaging should be ordered to rule out any structural causes.

4. Diagnostic studies could include lumbar x-rays to start. It would be appropriate to attempt a course of conservative measures prior to obtaining imaging. A lumbar x-ray would be the most appropriate radiographic study (at least PA and lateral views; oblique views would aid in diagnosis of facet arthropathy and flexion/extension view with listhesis). An MRI should be reserved for patients with neurologic deficits or symptoms, or for those with a high certainty of fracture, infection, cancer, or failure of conservative treatment.

5. Conservative measures such as ice, heat, massage, acupuncture, chiropractic/osteopathic manipulation, and/or physical therapy (manual treatment, modalities, core strengthening, and range of motion exercises) are first-line treatments. NSAIDs can relieve pain but should be used on a short-term basis if no contraindications (history of GERD, cardiovascular disease, or decreased kidney function). Opioids should be used short term only for severe pain and loss of function. Patient education and patient reassurance is important. This is a great opportunity to assure the patient his pain is likely to resolve and currently does not demonstrate any major serious concerns.

6. X-rays are indicated only for significant trauma or positive "red flags." You could start with a retrospective review of how often these guidelines are violated within your practice or clinic. Educate your colleagues and the patients on the guidelines and prospectively evaluate the impact. Continue with a

PDSA (plan, do, see, and act) cycle by adapting various educational techniques to see which is the most effective.

7. This is a great opportunity to educate the patient about opioid pain medications and the risks of starting/using such medication. He should understand the risks of misuse, dependence, abuse, and the reasons for attempting non-opioid alternatives first. There are guidelines that should be followed when considering opioids. Including, using the lowest dose possible, only prescribing what is needed for the situation, frequent reevaluation, documentation of functional benefits that validate the use of opioids, and potential urine drug screening to rule out the use of other controlled or illicit drugs that make prescribing opioids dangerous. In this particular situation, a prescription-strength anti-inflammatory and a muscle relaxant would be most appropriate with short-term follow-up.

BIBLIOGRAPHY

Chou R, Qaseem A, Snow V, et al. Diagnosis and treatment of low back pain: a joint clinical practice guideline from the American college of physicians and the American pain society. *Ann Intern Med.* 2007;147:478–491. https://doi.org/10.7326/0003-4819-147-7-200710020-00006

Traeger A, Buchbinder R, Harris I, et al. Diagnosis and management of low-back pain in primary care. *CMAJ.* November 13, 2017;189(45):E1386–E1395. https://doi.org/10.1503/cmaj.170527

14 Spinal Cord Injury

Argyrios Stampas and Joel Frontera

A 35-year-old man with traumatic cervical spinal cord injury sustained 5 years ago in a motor vehicle accident status post cervical decompression and fusion presents to your clinic with complaints of loss of hand function. His physical exam from last year was significant for C7 AIS C.

Questions

1. What more do you want to know about the patient's history, comorbidities, and social situation? Please tell me why you are asking for these specifics.

2. How would you go about performing a physical exam on this patient? Why are these maneuvers/exam components important?

The patient tells you that he has been having progressive loss of strength over 2 to 3 months in his bilateral hands, affecting his manual wheelchair propulsion over the past few months as well as his grip. He is also having hand and finger dysesthesias and neck pain that feels like soreness. He denies changes in bowel and bladder function and reports no falls or trauma. Physical exam is significant for C5 sensory level with C7 motor level. The motor exam has not changed significantly from prior exams. Tinel's and Phalen's tests are equivocal bilaterally.

3. What is the differential diagnosis for this patient? Tell me the most likely diagnosis and why.

4. What diagnostic test or tests would you order and why?

Cervical x-ray is negative for hardware failure and acute fracture, and MRI reveals no syrinx. Electromyography-nerve conduction study (EMG-NCS) is significant for median neuropathy at the wrist.

5. Outline the treatment plan. Please tell me the initial treatment and next steps if that fails.

Outpatient physical therapy was recommended for this patient, but he says that transportation is an issue as the mobility transportation system does not service his area. How would you address this issue with the patient?

6. What are the options for his rehabilitation?

Patient wants to know how did this happen. He thought his new wheelchair would help with this.

7. Explain to him how this situation arose.

Answers

1. Time period of occurrence. Would like to know about sensory changes in the upper extremities, changes with his bowel program (constipation, accidents, etc.), changes with his bladder program (frequency, urgency, urinary tract infections, etc.), history of recent fall or trauma, and changes with neuropathic pain and/or paresthesia. Specific information is needed regarding the hand function loss. Review of systems should include constitutional issues (fevers, chills, and weight loss/gain), polydipsia, hunger, fatigue, and blurred vision (type 2 diabetes mellitus [DMII] symptoms). This is important to document any neurological change that may be related to his spinal cord injury (SCI). The patient tells you that he has been having progressive loss of strength over 2 to 3 months in his bilateral hands, affecting his manual wheelchair propulsion over the past few months as well as his grip. He is also having hand and finger dysesthesias and neck pain that feels like soreness. He denies changes in bowel and bladder function and reports no falls or trauma. What is critical to do on physical exam?

2. Physical exam is significant for C5 sensory level with C7 motor level. The motor exam has not changed significantly from prior exams. Tinel's and Phalen's tests are equivocal bilaterally.

3. Differential diagnosis includes carpal tunnel syndrome, ulnar neuropathy, radiculopathy, hardware failure and cord/root impingement, syringomyelia, and peripheral neuropathy.

4. A cervical x-ray is indicated to rule out hardware failure, an MRI of the cervical spine to rule out syringomyelia, and a bilateral NCS/EMG to rule out radiculopathy.

5. Treatment includes occupational therapy consultation for learning to improve wrist positioning during activities of daily living and ergonomic wheelchair adjustments, education on ergonomic workspace, and wrist/hand orthosis to be worn while sleeping, Therapist referral should also include an evaluation for power-assist mobility for his manual wheelchair. He would also benefit from outpatient therapy for strengthening. Weight loss would also make wheelchair propulsion easier. Symptoms may improve with medications including gabapentin/pregabalin/amitriptyline/nortriptyline for neuropathic pain management. If he fails to improve with this, repeat NCS/EMG should be obtained to evaluate for worsening neuropathy. Corticosteroid injections can be considered. Surgery would be a last resort, especially since it might limit his ability to transfer independently during postoperative recovery.

6. He may well qualify for home therapies as he is homebound.

7. Unless properly measured and trained, the technique for manual wheelchair propulsion can lead to injuries to the arms and hands. A properly measured

custom wheelchair is half of the equation. The other half of the equation is to have a skilled therapist observe wheelchair propulsion techniques to ensure the lowest risk of harm to the upper body. Therefore, a referral to a skilled therapist, to ensure ergonomic techniques are incorporated in wheelchair propulsion as well as activities of daily living, will help reduce further injuries.

BIBLIOGRAPHY

Kentar Y, Zastrow R, Bradley H, et al. Prevalence of upper extremity pain in a population of people with paraplegia. *Spinal Cord.* 2018;56:695–703. https://doi.org/10.1038/s41393-018-0062-6

Tan W-H, Skelton F. *Overuse injuries in disorders of the central nervous system.* Knowledge NOW. 2013. http://me.aapmr.org/kn/article.html?id=28

A 35-year-old male presents to your clinic with C5 AIS C spinal cord injury complaining of worsening spasticity over the past year. The spasms interfere with his transfers and have caused him to fall several times. He is taking baclofen 20 mg four times daily and complains of fatigue from it.

Questions

1. What more do you want to know about the patient's history, comorbidities, and social situation? Please tell me why you are asking for these specifics.

2. How would you go about performing a physical exam on this patient? Why are these maneuvers/exam components important?

His exam is stable with C5 AIS C. He has stool in his rectum and has decreased bowel sounds with a distended abdomen. Spasticity is 3/4 on the Modified Ashworth Scale for shoulder, elbow flexors and finger flexors, hip adductors, knee extensors and flexors, and ankle plantar and dorsi-flexors. He has sustained clonus in upper and lower limbs.

3. What is the differential diagnosis for this patient? Tell me the most likely diagnosis and why.

4. What diagnostic test or tests would you order and why?

After a few minutes, the patient returns having completed an abdominal x-ray that is significant for a large volume of stool and nephrolithiasis.

5. Outline the treatment plan. Please tell me the initial treatment and next steps if that fails.

He returns to the clinic after successful lithotripsy and bowel cleanout. He continues to have spasticity for which he takes baclofen, and he is concerned about the side effects of constipation and sedation. You added tizanidine, which made him orthostatic, and tried dantrolene, but this made him feel weak all over. Patient is interested in discussing the option of an intrathecal baclofen pump.

6. What process is involved in setting this up?

Patient wants to go ahead with the implantation. He asks how the pump works and what side effects he may experience.

7. Describe the risks and benefits of the intrathecal baclofen pump to him.

Answers

1. Changes in spasticity can often result from noxious stimulants below the level of injury, similar to triggers for autonomic dysreflexia (AD). Therefore, a spinal cord specific review of systems is needed.
   - Neurologic: The patient has not had noticeable differences with his sensation or strength.
   - Neurogenic bladder: He has had more bladder accidents in between catheterizations.
   - Neurogenic bowel: He has had less production with his bowel program. Patient reports he has switched his bowel routine to every third day to make it easier on his caregiver.
   - Spasticity: Worsened per history. He has not noticed any new position changes that trigger spasticity, just that they are stronger and occurring more frequently at rest.
   - Skin: Intact, with no pressure injuries.
   - Pain: He thinks he might have more low back pain. He denies worsened neck pain.

2. An evaluation of his neurologic function is important to assess for causes such as a syrinx. Performing a comprehensive International Standards for Neurological Classification of Spinal Cord Injury (ISCNSCI) is important to pinpoint a change in his neurologic level. An assessment of his tone with Modified Ashworth Scale is essential as well as evaluating any other noxious stimuli that may be causing the increased spasms such as ingrown toenail, skin pressure injury, constipation via abdominal exam, and so on.

3. Any noxious stimuli, from urine retention, constipation, and bowel obstruction, to skin injuries, can cause an increase in spasticity. In the setting of other neurologic findings, a syrinx should also be considered. In this case, highest on the differential is constipation with large stool burden. Bladder, bowel, and skin problems are the most common causes for worsening spasticity.

4. Urinalysis with culture is ordered to rule out urinary tract infection. Abdominal x-ray is ordered to evaluate stool burden.

5. Aggressive bowel cleanout (magnesium citrate, lactulose, or high volume polyethylene glycol) and Fleet enema to reduce stool burden are the next steps. After bowel cleanout, the routine bowel program needs to be upgraded. A urologist follow-up for nephrolithiasis is recommended. Add tizanidine and/or dantrolene for his spasticity. Tizanidine can lower blood pressure (BP), so it is not indicated in hypotension. Dantrolene is contraindicated in hepatic impairment, so liver function tests need to be obtained prior to initiation. If symptoms persist would consider an MRI of the cervical spine to rule out a syrinx.

6. He will need to have a trial dose intrathecally to see how he responds. Depending on the institution, this may be performed by either the physiatrist or the implanting surgeon. In either case, he will need a physical therapy evaluation prior to the trial dose and another 4 to 6 hours after the dose is given.

7. The pump delivers the medicine directly to the fluid around the spinal cord, requiring a much smaller dose and subsequently fewer systemic side effects. There is a risk of infection and meningitis with the surgical pump implantation. There are also postoperative restrictions to range of motion (ROM), which may require further assistance from caregivers for several weeks. Maintenance of the pump requires physician visits for pump refills several times per year. Compliance with pump refills is imperative. We would need to explain the risk of sudden withdrawal if the pump is not refilled or the system fails. Stress the importance of follow-up and close monitoring of symptoms of withdrawal or overdose.

BIBLIOGRAPHY

Adams MM, Hicks AL. Spasticity after spinal cord injury. *Spinal Cord.* 2005;43:577–586. https://doi.org/10.1038/sj.sc.3101757

Francisco GE. The role of intrathecal baclofen therapy in the upper motor neuron syndrome. *Eur Med Phys.* 2004;40:131–143.

Kaila A. Holtz KA, Lipson R, Noonan VK, et al. Prevalence and effect of problematic spasticity after traumatic spinal cord injury. *Arch Phys Med Rehabil.* June 2017;98(6):1132–1138. https://doi.org/10.1016/j.apmr.2016.09.124

A 56-year-old male presents to your clinic complaining of worsened weakness since his back surgery 3 weeks ago. He tells you that it was the third surgery on his lower back, and he needed it because he was getting weak in his legs.

Questions

1. What more do you want to know about the patient's history, comorbidities, and social situation? Please tell me why you are asking for these specifics.

2. How would you go about performing a physical exam on this patient? Why are these maneuvers/exam components important?

Physical exam is significant for 4/5 strength in L2 and L3 and 1/5 strength in L4-S1 myotomes, reduced sensation in L2-S5 dermatomes, 1+ patellar reflexes and areflexic in Achilles reflex, positive deep anal pressure, no voluntary anal contraction, and no anal wink with pinprick.

3. What is the differential diagnosis for this patient? Tell me the most likely diagnosis and why.

4. What diagnostic test or tests would you order and why?

MRI show an area of hematoma formation at L3-L4

5. Outline the treatment plan. Please tell me the initial treatment and next steps if that fails.

Patient calls you saying that he has made great progress in rehabilitation but still has bowel and bladder dysfunction. Insurance will not accept an extension on his stay, and he is scheduled to be discharged tomorrow. He wants some help as he does not know how to be independent with management of his bowel and bladder.

6. How would you advocate for him?

He has followed your program and has not had bowel or bladder accidents. However, he is concerned about his sexual function and wants to know what can be expected with treatment, if possible.

7. What do you advise him about this?

Answers

1. Would want to know about his prior surgeries, the indication, and his outcome. He is not a good historian but tells you that he had two minor back surgeries for back pain because of a disc problem and that they did not work so he had to have this last operation. The back pain worsened, and he was developing weakness in his legs and catching his foot and tripping at times. He tells you that his operation was on L2 and L3. A lumbar spine x-ray suggested degenerative disc disease and spondylosis. An MRI showed disc disease and herniation at the L2-L3 level. EMG was significant for bilateral L3 radiculopathy. He had an uncomplicated surgery. Postoperatively he had profound weakness in his feet that somewhat improved with high-dose steroids. He had an indwelling catheter that was removed on day of discharge and, after a long time, he voided about 1 L of urine. He is now often incontinent of bowel and bladder.

2. Critical components of the physical exam are manual motor testing in the bilateral lower extremities (BLE), sensory testing in the BLE, deep tendon reflexes in the bilateral upper extremities (BUE) and BLE, rectal exam with pin and light touch, and observation of anal wink reflex. We should also inquire about changes in bowel and bladder habits.

3. The differential diagnosis assessment is a possible conus medullaris syndrome or cauda equina syndrome with lower motor neuron bowel and bladder. Due to his history of surgery in the lumbar region and findings on physical exam, an injury to the conus or cauda equina is possible. The reasons for injury include iatrogenic at the time of surgery versus postoperative complications including infection or hematoma.

4. A diagnostic test that should be considered is a repeat MRI to assess for possible issues with surgery including a hematoma, loose hardware, or nerve impingement. Because of the broad differential including infection, MRI with and without contrast is recommended. This should most likely be treated as an emergency.

5. Patient should immediately seek a neurosurgical consultation, ideally from his last surgeon. Neurosurgery performed an evacuation of the hematoma. The patient had improvement of weakness symptoms but continues to have bowel and bladder incontinence. Because of his bowel and bladder incontinence, as well as his mobility impairments, he was referred and admitted to acute inpatient rehabilitation.

6. An important aspect of any inpatient program for a person with spinal cord injury is the education and training of long-term bowel and bladder care. A comprehensive program in which the patient trains with nursing staff to become independent should be a priority. He should have a bowel program with promotility (senna, bisacodyl) and bulking (fiber) with an enema

or manual disempaction for daily bowel movements. Similarly, bladder management should maintain hygiene with scheduled emptying of safe urine volumes. Because continence was not achieved, there may be an opportunity to have an extension of his rehabilitation admission. However, there are a multitude of factors that can interfere with achieving continence of bowel and bladder function, some of which would not improve with an extended admission. However, understanding the proper techniques of bowel and bladder management can help continue training toward independence as an outpatient. Close follow-up with his physician as an outpatient would be recommended.

7. When discussing sexuality, rapport should be established. In this case, rapport has been established and both patient and physician are comfortable talking about sex and sexuality. In incomplete injuries, as in this case, erection can occur both psychogenically and reflexively in the vast majority of cases. Sildenafil (Viagra) can help with erectile dysfunction if rigidity cannot be maintained during intercourse. As far as ejaculation, the majority of patients with incomplete injuries regain this function. There are no Food and Drug Administration (FDA)-approved medications for ejaculation disorders due to neurologic conditions. Medications and alcohol can impair ejaculation, including antidepressants and BP medications. However, orgasm can still be achieved. Regarding fertility, specialized clinics can harvest sperm successfully for this purpose.

BIBLIOGRAPHY

Gonzalez-Fernandez M. Bowel care medications. In: Gonzalez-Fernandez M, Friedman JD, eds. *Physical Medicine and Rehabilitation Pocket Companion*. Vol 1. 1st ed. Demos; 2011:326–329.

Hadiji N, Mieusset R, Previnaire JG, et al. Ejaculation and sperm characteristics in men with cauda equina and conus medullaris syndromes. *Spinal Cord*. 2017;55:612–617. https://doi.org/10.1038/sc.2017.5

Podnar S, Trsinar B, Vodusek DB. Bladder dysfunction in patients with cauda equina lesions. *Neurourol Urodyn*. 2006;25(1):23–31. https://doi.org/10.1002/nau.20188

Todd NV, Dickson RA. Standards of care in cauda equina syndrome. *Br J Neurosurg*. October 2016;30(5):518–522. https://doi.org/10.1080/02688697.2016.1187254

A 35-year-old male with C5 AIS A tetraplegia sustained in a motor vehicle collision 2 weeks ago is admitted to your spinal cord unit at a free-standing rehabilitation hospital. He has a tracheostomy and is on a ventilator at night, with intravenous (IV) access in his right arm, and an indwelling Foley catheter. Nursing calls you immediately because of complaints of headache, flushing, and chills.

Questions

1. What more do you want to know about the patient's history, comorbidities, and social situation? Please tell me why you are asking for these specifics.

2. How would you go about performing a physical exam on this patient? Why are these maneuvers/exam components important?

His systolic BP is 150/95 mmHg, and pulse is 55. Otherwise, vitals are within normal limits. His Foley is not draining.

3. What is the differential diagnosis for this patient? Tell me the most likely diagnosis and why.

4. What diagnostic test or tests would you order and why?

Patient feels much better but now is very concerned about what he just experienced.

5. Outline the treatment plan. Please tell me the initial treatment and next steps if that fails

He has another episode of autonomic dysreflexia a week later. His systolic BP is now 180 mmHg. You discover an edematous, erythematous, ingrown toenail. There is no podiatrist available at your hospital, and you most likely will need to send patient out to her clinic tomorrow afternoon.

6. How can care be facilitated?

He returns to your outpatient clinic with his wife 1 month after discharge. He tells you that he does not consistently get his bowel program because his wife works during the day, and his teenage daughter is not comfortable doing it. He gets autonomic dysreflexia once or twice a week due to constipation.

7. Discuss with them how the bowel program might be facilitated.

Answers

1. Check vital signs (BP, temperature, heart rate, respiration rate, pulse oximetry), penis, drainage of Foley, and any pressure on the skin from clothing, sheets, or orthotics. Given his level of injury and severity AIS A, AD is on top of the differential. Systolic BP over 20 mmHg from baseline causes the symptoms of AD, which describe the patient's symptoms.

2. Patient should be checked from top to bottom to see if there are any noxious stimuli on the skin, including pressure from adducted knees, tangled sheets or clothing, or even a limb pressed against the side of the bed. Ingrown toenails can cause this as well. The penis should be inspected for trauma, and the indwelling catheter must be draining. One should do a rectal exam to exclude fecal impaction (done with lidocaine gel), the anal sphincter should be inspected for hemorrhoids or anal fissures, and the sacrum should be evaluated for pressure injuries. After thorough inspection, the patient should be put into a more upright, seated position. BP cuff should be applied monitoring. Loosen clothing and flush the Foley.

3. The highest on the differential is AD due to bladder overdistention from catheter obstruction. This can explain all of his symptoms. Lower on the differential include a migraine headache, which can cause pain and increased BP as a normal sympathetic response to pain, however it should not cause flushing or chills. Other diagnoses to consider are an infectious process or a pulmonary process.

4. Infection must be ruled out, therefore a complete blood count (CBC) should be ordered. Electrolyte disturbances, renal function, and liver function may impact treatment, therefore a comprehensive metabolic panel (CMP) should be ordered. Blood pressures should be checked every 5 minutes. Pulse oximetry can help rule out any respiratory compromise. If there is a concern of respiratory compromise, a STAT chest x-ray would be needed.

5. You need to educate the family using lay terms. Explain how the spinal cord injury affects internal organs in addition to the arms and legs. AD can cause elevated BP that leads to seizures, retinal hemorrhage, pulmonary edema, renal insufficiency, myocardial infarction, cerebral hemorrhage, and death. You need to explain the early warning signs such as flushing, sweating, and headache. You need to discuss how problems with bowel, bladder, and skin care are the three main causes of AD.

6. Hold from therapy until BP is controlled; monitor vitals q2 hours, and administer analgesics, topical or oral. Use fast-acting antihypertensive medications to control BP (nitro paste, nitroglycerine sublingual, hydralazine, nifedipine, or captopril). Working with hospital administration to address the issue of hospital consultants as it could become a patient access issue, which could delay treatment. This may include paying for transport to specialist's offices when patient does not have privileges at your hospital.

7. Stress the importance of the bowel program for his medical condition. Ask them if it would be easier to perform the bowel program after the wife gets home from work. In some states, Medicaid will provide home health aides for several hours per day. Sometimes private insurance will provide this as well. Usually this is quite limited under Medicare. He may have to hire help. The inclusion of a social worker in the outpatient setting is essential to navigate some lapses in care. The importance of identifying a care provider should be part of the rehabilitation discharge planning and establishing tasks with providers. Surgical management options exist, such as a colostomy, which can greatly improve the quality of life of people who cannot otherwise perform their bowel program independently.

BIBLIOGRAPHY

Christopher and Dana Reeve Foundation. *Autonomic dysreflexia pamphlets.* http://www.christopherreeve.org/site/c.mtKZKgMWKwG/b.4453413/k.5E2A/Autonomic_Dysreflexia.htm

Garstang SV, Walker H. Cardiovascular and autonomic dysfunctions after spinal cord injury. In: Kirshblum S, Campagnolo DI, eds. *Spinal Cord Medicine.* 2nd ed. Wolters Kluwer Health/Lippincott Williams & Wilkins; 2011.

Kirshblum S, Eren F, Solinsky R, et al. Diastolic blood pressure changes during episodes of autonomic dysreflexia. *J of Spinal Cord Med.* 2020. https://doi.org/10.1080/10790268.2020.1757273

Krassioukov A, Warburton DE, Teasell R, et al. A systematic review of the management of autonomic dysreflexia after spinal cord injury. *Arch Phys Med Rehabil.* 2009;90(4):682–695. https://doi.org/10.1016/j.apmr.2008.10.017

You see an 85-year-old woman with a 3-month history of central cord syndrome in a skilled nursing facility. She sustained a nonoperative spinal injury. She was wearing a Halo vest previously but the spine surgeon transitioned to a less restrictive brace, the sternal occipital mandibular immobilizer (SOMI) 2 weeks ago, due to pin site migration.

Questions

1. What more do you want to know about the patient's history, comorbidities, and social situation? Please tell me why you are asking for these specifics.

2. How would you go about performing a physical exam on this patient? Why are these maneuvers/exam components important?

You found the patient has a deep tissue injury on the occipital area that is draining serosanguinous fluid. Patient denies any fever or chills.

3. What is the differential diagnosis for this patient? Tell me the most likely diagnosis and why.

4. What diagnostic test or tests would you order and why?

The pressure sore is a stage 2. The head CT did not show osteomyelitis, and CBC and C-reactive protein (CRP) were within normal limits.

5. Outline the treatment plan. Please tell me the initial treatment and next steps if that fails

You are concerned about how the skilled nursing facility did not notice the pressure sore developing.

6. How would you approach a quality improvement program to assure that this does not happen again?

The patient's son calls you and he is very disturbed about how this happened. He is threatening legal action against the facility.

7. How would you resolve this conflict?

Answers

1. Her rehabilitation course was uneventful, and she was discharged to a skilled nursing facility. The Halo vest was removed by the spine surgeon 2 weeks ago, and she is now wearing a hard cervical thoracic orthotic (SOMI) brace. She tells you she has pain on the back of her head from the brace.

2. Pertinent exam findings include skin exam. Transition her to a bed to examine her skin closely while maintaining stability. Repeat her neurological exam.

3. Differential diagnosis includes a pressure injury secondary to bracing, skin abscess, or trauma. Given the history of a change in bracing leading to redness of the skin at a point of contact, pressure injury is highest on the list.

4. CT head to rule out the possibility of an underlying osteomyelitis, as well as CBC, CRP, or erythrocyte sedimentation rate (ESR) for signs of infection given wound drainage.

5. You call the orthoptist to make the proper adjustments on the collar and educate the patient about pressure relief. Wound care should be ordered for monitoring and dressing changes. With continued pressure, the occipital wound will not heal. Other than the HALO, all of the appropriate braces that restrict ROM can apply pressure to the occiput. If she does not wear a brace, she risks further spinal cord injury from spine instability, until her spine heals. If the sore does not heal, you may need to have the neurosurgeon reinstall a HALO.

6. You should form an interprofessional team to address the issue including nursing and the orthotist. Develop a policy for the daily monitoring for skin breakdown in patients in SOMI braces. Put together an educational session for members of the nursing staff about safe removal of the brace for this purpose.

7. It is critical to be honest with him and to explain all the facts. Tell him that this is a common complication of the SOMI brace and explain the treatment plan. In most cases, this is very treatable, but sometimes a HALO brace has to be reinitiated. In the meantime, also let the facility know of the son's concerns so that they can address these concerns as well.

BIBLIOGRAPHY

American Spinal Injury Association. *International Standards for Neurological and Functional Classification of Spinal Cord Injury—Revised 2011.* ASIA; 2011.

Devivo MJ, Chen Y. Trends in new injuries, prevalent cases and aging with spinal cord injury. *Arch Phys Med Rehabil.* 2011;92(3):332–338. https://doi.org/10.1016/j.apmr.2010.08.031

Yang J, Gosai E, Avers S. *Cervical, thoracic and lumbosacral orthoses.* Knowledge NOW. 2017. https://now.aapmr.org/cervical-thoracic-and-lumbosacral-orthoses

15 Sports Medicine

Brian J. Krabak, Brian C. Liem, Melinda S. Loveless, and Amanda Wise

CASE 1

A 53-year-old female recreational softball player presents to your sports clinic with a 6-month history of left shoulder pain and limited range of motion (ROM).

Questions

1. What more do you want to know about the patient's history, comorbidities, and social situation? Please tell me why you are asking for these specifics.

2. How would you go about performing a physical exam on this patient? Why are these maneuvers/exam components important?

She tells you that the pain developed insidiously without trauma. Location is mainly in the anterior shoulder but can radiate all the way to her wrist. Pain is worsened with reaching in any direction, and she is especially limited in her ability to reach overhead or behind her back. This loss of ROM interferes with dressing and bathing, and pain interrupts her sleep. Cervical motion has no effect on her pain. The patient has a normal neurologic examination but significant restrictions in both active and passive ROM of the shoulder in all planes but especially with external rotation and abduction. She has pain with Hawkin's and Neer's maneuvers but a negative empty can test. Her cervical ROM is full without reproduction of typical pain. Spurling's maneuver is negative.

3. What is the differential diagnosis for this patient? Tell me the most likely diagnosis and why.

4. What diagnostic test or tests would you order and why?

X-ray and ultrasound of the shoulder are normal. Authorization for MRI was denied by the insurance company.

5. Outline the treatment plan. Please tell me the initial treatment and next steps if that fails.

She works as a receptionist in a dental office. She asks whether this condition is work related and if she can make a workers' compensation claim.

6. How should you respond?

The patient states that she has read online about "tendinosis" and wonders if she could also have this.

7. Tell me in lay terms how you would describe "tendinosis."

Answers

1. Key history elements
   - Onset (insidious or traumatic): Traumatic onset may lead you more to conditions such as acromioclavicular (AC) separation, fracture, or full-thickness rotator cuff tears
   - Main location of pain (anterior lateral shoulder, superior shoulder, scapular region). Location helps to determine which structures may be involved (AC joint, posterior rotator cuff, biceps tendon)
   - Exacerbating factors (reaching overhead, behind), alleviating factors, any associated pain sleeping on the shoulder at night (common symptom of rotator cuff pathology)
   - Functional limitations (gives a sense of how bothersome the pain is and how aggressive treatments need to be)
   - Any symptoms worsened with cervical motion (to assess possible cervical source for pain)
   - Underlying diabetes or thyroid disorders that can predispose the patient to conditions such as adhesive capsulitis

2. Essential examination elements include active and passive shoulder ROM, assessment of upper extremity strength, sensation, reflexes, presence of painful arc (60–120 degrees shoulder abduction) that is seen in rotator cuff impingement, special shoulder tests (Hawkin's, Neer's, empty can; Figure 15.1), palpation of shoulder structures for tenderness (AC joint, biceps tendon, subacromial region, upper trapezius for trigger points), and cervical ROM and Spurling's maneuver for cervical radiculitis.

3. Differential diagnosis includes rotator cuff impingement/tear, adhesive capsulitis (frozen shoulder), and glenohumeral osteoarthritis. The patient likely has adhesive capsulitis. Patients with adhesive capsulitis generally present with restrictions in both active **and** passive ROM, as opposed to rotator cuff disease where active ROM is restricted but passive ROM is approximately normal. Glenohumeral osteoarthritis can present with both passive and active ROM and can be evaluated with x-rays.

4. Tests should include x-rays with the following views—anteroposterior (AP), Grashey, and axillary to rule out glenohumeral osteoarthritis. Ultrasound of the shoulder may show rotator cuff tears or tendinosis. An MRI may also be considered to rule out full-thickness rotator cuff tears if there is a history of trauma (these might require surgery) but is not necessary for the diagnosis of adhesive capsulitis. In general, there are no pathognomonic signs on MRI for adhesive capsulitis. It is a clinical diagnosis.

5. Initial treatment consists of education of the natural history of adhesive capsulitis, which in most cases resolves over 1 to 2 years. Treatment includes physical therapy focused on improving function, pain control, ROM, and scapular and rotator cuff strengthening. Oral analgesics for pain should be prescribed, usually nonsteroidals if no contraindications. Acetaminophen can also be considered. If there is no response to initial treatment, then intra-articular

injections of steroid or hydrodilation with large volumes of normal saline can be beneficial for pain. While most interventions have not been found to change the natural history, there is some suggestion that steroids may help shorten duration of symptoms (Redler 2019). Manipulation under anesthesia and arthroscopic capsular release is typically reserved for refractory cases greater than 6 months (Hsu 2011).

6. Obtain a thorough history of details of her job. A receptionist generally does not have excessive use of her shoulder to explain this. The patient's condition likely is covered by medical insurance but not workers' compensation (aka Labor and Industries). She can receive unpaid time off from work for therapies or doctors' appointments under the Family Medical Leave Act (FMLA).

7. Acknowledge that the patient may indeed have tendinosis in addition to adhesive capsulitis. Tendinosis can be thought of as a "wear and tear" of a tendon. With regard to the shoulder, tendinosis can be seen mainly in the rotator cuff. An analogy to a tendon is a piece of twine/rope. The individual fibers of the twine are similar to the collagen fibers that make up a tendon. If there is sufficient "tug and pull" on the tendon from repetitive motion, the fibers can separate, causing overall thickening of the twine with gaps in between, which are analogous to cuff microtears. An ultrasound can help evaluate for this but clinically, her presentation is most consistent with adhesive capsulitis.

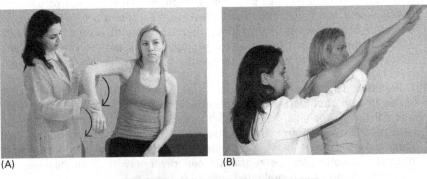

(A) (B)

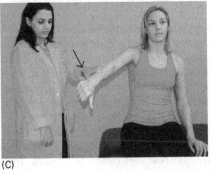

(C)

Figure 15.1 (A) Hawkin's, (B) Neer's, and (C) empty can tests.

BIBLIOGRAPHY

Hsu JE, Anakwenze OA, Warrender WJ, et al. Current review of adhesive capsulitis. *J Shoulder Elbow Surg.* 2011;20(3):502–514. https://doi.org/10.1016/j.jse.2010.08.023

Kingston K, Curry EJ, Galvin JW, et al. Shoulder adhesive capsulitis: epidemiology and predictors of surgery. *J Shoulder Elbow Surg.* 2018;27(8):1437–1443. https://doi.org/10.1016/j.jse.2018.04.004

Ramirez J. Adhesive capsulitis: diagnosis and management. *Am Fam Physician.* 2019;99(5):297–300.

Redler LH, Dennis ER. Treatment of adhesive capsulitis of the shoulder. *J Am Acad Orthop Surg.* 2019;27(12):e544–e554. https://doi.org/10.5435/JAAOS-D-17-00606

An 18-year-old male college football player presents to your office with complaints of right shoulder pain and weakness after playing in a game last evening.

Questions

1. What more do you want to know about the patient's history, comorbidities, and social situation? Please tell me why you are asking for these specifics.

2. How would you go about performing a physical exam on this patient? Why are these maneuvers/exam components important?

He tells you that he fell backward on his outstretched arm and felt that his shoulder "popped out" but was able to later "pop it back in" after a maneuver by the team's athletic trainer. He now has difficulty elevating his arm to comb his hair. Examination reveals partial weakness of right shoulder abduction and shoulder external rotation and a well-circumscribed area of decreased sensation over the lateral shoulder. He has minimal discomfort with Hawkin's and Neer's maneuvers. Speed's and empty can maneuvers are negative. Cervical ROM is normal without pain and Spurling's maneuver is negative.

3. What is the differential diagnosis for this patient? Tell me the most likely diagnosis and why.

4. What diagnostic test or tests would you order and why?

X-ray and MRI of the shoulder demonstrate a Hill-Sachs lesion but normal rotator cuff tendons and labrum. X-ray and MRI of the cervical spine are normal. No ultrasound available. Electromyography (EMG)/nerve conduction study (NCS): Axillary motor NCS demonstrate normal distal latency but decreased amplitude. Needle EMG demonstrated the presence of fibrillation potentials in the deltoid and teres minor muscles. Motor unit analysis of these muscles demonstrated decreased motor recruitment. All other muscles tested were normal.

5. Outline the treatment plan. Please tell me the initial treatment and next steps if that fails.

He has a big game next week against his school's biggest rivals and wants to know if he will be ready to play.

6. How do you counsel him?

He asks about what it means to have nerve injury. "Will I be paralyzed?"

7. Explain his injury to him in lay terms.

Answers

1. Key history elements
   - Onset (traumatic or nontraumatic): Details of any trauma preceding the onset of symptoms are key. Did he fall on an outstretched and externally rotated arm (shoulder dislocation)? Direct fall on the shoulder (AC joint injury)? Depression of shoulder while neck laterally rotated (stinger/burner)? If there has been no trauma, pain and weakness could still indicate a shoulder ethology (rotator cuff impingement, partial tear) but could also be from a cervical disc herniation (often these are not preceded by any trauma).
   - Is there presence of neck pain, numbness/tingling, or weakness (suggestive of cervical etiology)?
   - Exact motion of weakness (abduction, forward flexion, internal or external rotation). A pattern of certain weakness might be more suggestive of a myotomal versus peripheral nerve (suprascapular, axillary) etiology versus isolated tendon/muscle involvement (biceps tendon, supraspinatus tendon).

2. Essential examination elements include active and passive shoulder ROM, upper extremity strength (especially external rotation), sensation, reflexes, palpation of shoulder structures (AC joint, clavicle, subacromial region, upper trap and periscapular muscles), special shoulder tests (Speed's for biceps tendinopathy, O'Brien's for labral tear, Hawkin's, Neer's for impingement, empty can for supraspinatus tendinopathy), cervical spine ROM, and Spurling's maneuver.

3. The presence of weakness on exam suggests neurologic compromise, so differential diagnosis includes C5 to C6 radiculopathy, brachial plexopathy (upper trunk), and shoulder dislocation with axillary nerve injury and suprascapular neuropathy. However, weakness can also be secondary to pain from an injury to bone/joint (fracture humeral head) or tendon (supraspinatus and infraspinatus tear). The most likely diagnosis in this case is injury to the axillary nerve after shoulder dislocation.

4. Diagnostic testing includes x-rays of the shoulder and cervical spine to evaluate for fracture, MRI of the shoulder to evaluate for rotator cuff tear (supraspinatus) and signs of anterior shoulder dislocation (Hill Sachs lesion [Figure 15.2], Bankart lesion), and cervical spine to evaluate for cervical nerve root impingement. Ultrasound can also evaluate for rotator cuff tear. Electrodiagnostic studies to evaluate for peripheral nerve injury versus brachial plexopathy versus radiculopathy.

5. Treatments include a sling for comfort for a few days and rest from sport to allow the axillary nerve to recover. Physical therapy is helpful to strengthen shoulder abductors, dynamic shoulder stabilizers (rotator cuff and biceps tendon), and scapular stabilizers. Oral analgesics help with pain associated with capsular sprain from the dislocation but not nerve recovery.

6. Unfortunately, it is highly unlikely that he will be ready to play in the game next week. In order to return to play, he will require full pain-free shoulder ROM and strength before advancing to sport-specific drills and then contact practice. This can take weeks and the best treatment is to ensure he has proper rest to allow the axillary nerve to recover and gradually progress his rehabilitation to prevent further reinjury.

7. You need to explain his injury in lay terms. He has injured his axillary nerve. He has decreased but some recruitment (muscle activity) on electrodiagnostic studies that is suggestive of a good prognosis for recovery. This means that the nerve is still working, but has mild damage. There is no indication that he will be "paralyzed" or have long-term functional limitations. The nerve should recover over the next month or 2 but he should be closely monitored in follow-up visits.

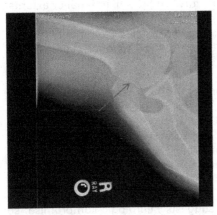

X-ray—Axillary

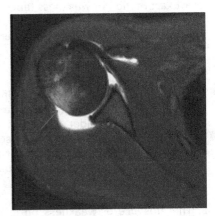

MRI—Axillary view

Figure 15.2 Hill Sach's lesion.

BIBLIOGRAPHY

Atef A, El-Tantawy A, Gad H, et al. Prevalence of associated injuries after anterior shoulder dislocation: a prospective study. *Int Orthop*. 2016;40(3):519–524. https://doi.org/10.1007/s00264-015-2862-z

Robinson CM, Shur N, Sharpe T, et al. Injuries associated with traumatic anterior glenohumeral dislocations. *J Bone Joint Surg Am*. 2012;94(1):18–26. https://doi.org/10.2106/JBJS.J.01795

Watson S, Allen B, Grant JA. A clinical review of return-to-play considerations after anterior shoulder dislocation. *Sports Health*. 2016;8(4):336–341. https://doi.org/10.1177/1941738116651956

A 29-year-old male soccer player presents to your sports clinic with a 1-week history of left shoulder pain.

Questions

1. What more do you want to know about the patient's history, comorbidities, and social situation? Please tell me why you are asking for these specifics?

2. How would you go about performing a physical exam on this patient? Why are these maneuvers/exam components important?

He reports that his pain began after a fall onto the shoulder during a soccer game. He was able to get up from the fall and play through it but it has continued to bother him. Location is mainly in superior shoulder with some radiation into the upper trap. Pain is worsened when reaching overhead and across his body. There is associated clicking with shoulder movement but he has not noted any significant loss of ROM nor interruption in sleep. There is slight deformity of the AC joint but no bruising. The patient has a normal neurologic examination and full active and passive ROM of the shoulder. He has excellent strength with all rotator cuff testing. He has pain with cross-arm adduction and O'Brien's but a negative Hawkin's and empty can test. No reproduction of pain with cervical motion. Spurling's maneuver is negative.

3. What is the differential diagnosis for this patient? Tell me the most likely diagnosis and why.

4. What diagnostic test or tests would you order and why?

X-ray of bilateral AC joints demonstrates widening of the right AC joint and coracoclavicular (CC) interval (Figure 15.3) that is approximately 60% of the asymptomatic contralateral side. No fractures. Axillary view is normal. Ultrasound demonstrates normal rotator cuff tendons.

5. Outline the treatment plan. Please tell me the initial treatment and next steps if that fails.

After describing your diagnosis and treatment plan, the patient requests an MRI to "diagnose" the problem.

6. How should you respond?

The patient has heard about "cortisone" injections and would like to know if this helps his injury "heal."

7. How would you discuss this with him?

Answers

1. Key history elements:
   - Onset (insidious or traumatic): Traumatic onset may lead you more to conditions such as AC separation, fracture, or full-thickness rotator cuff tears.
   - Main location of pain (anterior lateral shoulder, superior shoulder, scapular region). Location helps to determine which structures may be involved (AC joint is typically over joint and superior shoulder, posterior rotator cuff, anterior for biceps tendon or anterior fibers of supraspinatus tendon).
   - Exacerbating factors (reaching overhead, behind), alleviating factors, any associated pain sleeping on the shoulder at night time (common symptom of rotator cuff pathology).
   - Functional limitations (gives a sense of how bothersome the pain is and what treatments may be needed).
   - Any symptoms worsened with cervical motion (to assess possible cervical source for pain).

2. Essential examination elements include active and passive shoulder ROM, assessment of upper extremity strength, sensation, reflexes, presence of painful arc (60–120 degrees shoulder abduction) that is seen in rotator cuff impingement, special shoulder tests (Cross-body adduction for AC joint; O'Brien's for AC joint for labral tear; Hawkin's; Neer's for impingement; empty can; palpation of shoulder structures for tenderness [AC joint, biceps tendon, subacromial region, upper trapezius for trigger points]), and cervical ROM and Spurling's maneuver (for cervical radiculitis; Figure 15.1).

3. Differential diagnosis includes AC joint injury (separation), greater tuberosity fracture, distal clavicle fracture, or rotator cuff impingement/tear. This patient likely has a Grade 3 AC joint injury. Patients with AC joint injury generally present with pain in the superior shoulder, tenderness over the AC joint, and pain with cross-body adduction. There are typically six types of AC joint injuries based on the Rockwood Classification.

4. Tests should include bilateral AC joint x-rays to compare the symptomatic AC and CC intervals to the asymptomatic side and to rule out distal clavicle fractures, and axillary views to evaluate for posterior clavicle displacement (grade V injuries) (Figure 15.3). Ultrasound of the shoulder may demonstrate an effusion of the joint and rule out rotator cuff pathology (Figure 15.4). An MRI is typically not necessary.

5. For grades 1 to 2 AC joint injuries, treatment is nonoperative. Treatment for grade 3 is controversial but can be treated nonoperatively if the patient has good strength and ROM. Initial treatment consists of a sling for comfort for up to 2 weeks. The patient can then be progressed to home exercises or formal physical therapy focused on improving function, pain control, ROM, and scapular and rotator cuff strengthening. Oral or topical analgesics can be prescribed for pain (topical diclofenac gel). Intra-articular injections of steroids can be considered after 3 months if there is still persistent pain.

6. Describe to the patient that an MRI is not typically needed to diagnose AC joint injuries and that x-rays provide sufficient evaluation of this condition. Explain that even if the MRI confirms an AC joint injury, based on the x-rays, a Grade 3 injury treatment would not necessarily change. MRI may be helpful to evaluate for other shoulder conditions but based on his history of falling onto his shoulder, excellent strength with rotator cuff testing, and negative empty can test, it is unlikely that there is a major rotator cuff (which is the biggest indication for earlier surgical intervention).

7. Cortisone or steroid injections are frequently used to treat painful conditions, but there are potential side effects (articular cartilage toxicity, immunosuppression). Their main effects are anti-inflammatory, and they also inhibit painful C-fibers. In many acute conditions, they are avoided given their potential to inhibit healing. Therefore, they can be helpful for pain but do not necessarily help a condition heal quicker, nor would steroids realign the joint.

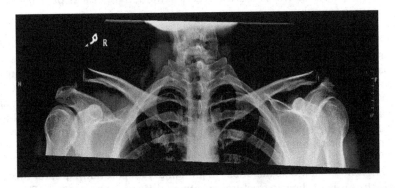

Figure 15.3 Acromioclavicular joint separation.

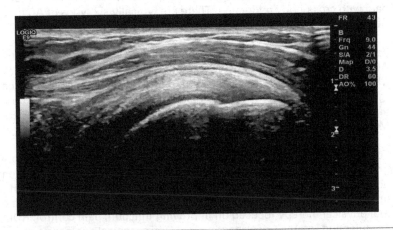

Figure 15.4 Ultrasound showing no effusion or rotator cuff tear.

BIBLIOGRAPHY

Frank RM, Cotter EJ, Leroux TS, et al. Acromioclavicular joint injuries: evidence-based treatment. *J Am Acad Orthop Surg.* 2019;27(17):e775–e788. https://doi.org/10.5435/JAAOS-D-17-00105

Stucken C, Cohen SB. Management of acromioclavicular joint injuries. *Orthop Clin North Am.* 2015;46(1):57–66. https://doi.org/10.1016/j.ocl.2014.09.003

CASE 4

A 14-year-old nationally ranked female gymnast presents with complaints of right knee pain for 7 days. She began practicing new tumbling passes 2 weeks earlier. She is scheduled to compete in a national competition in 3 weeks. Past medical history is unremarkable.

Questions

1. What key elements do you want to know from her history?

2. How would you perform a physical exam on this patient? What exam components and special tests are critical to do and why?

She notes she has pain along the medial femoral condyle and joint line. Symptoms worsen when landing any jumps. She has no history of stress fractures, significant weight loss, or amenorrhea. Examination reveals normal alignment and ROM. She has normal strength, sensation, and reflexes except for gluteus medius weakness on the right. She is tender to palpation over the right medial femoral condyle. She has no instability of the knee joint. McMurray's reproduces mild medial joint line pain, but no palpable click. She has pain with single-leg hop.

3. What is the differential diagnosis? Which is the most likely diagnosis and why?

4. What diagnostic testing, if any, is indicated?

X-rays of the right knee are normal. MRI of the knee reveals marrow edema involving the right medial femoral condyle. She is diagnosed with a medial femoral stress fracture.

5. Outline the treatment plan. What interventions would you recommend?

The patient is upset about her diagnosis and wants to know if the fracture will prevent her from being a collegiate athlete in the future.

6. How should you respond?

The patient wants to know what a "stress" fracture means.

7. Explain a stress fracture in lay terms.

Answers

1. The history should include a comprehensive, but focused evaluation of a knee injury. In this case, the symptoms appear to be due to an overuse injury, which should shape your specific questions. The history should include characterizing the pain, localization of pain, provocative and alleviating maneuvers, constitutional symptoms, and a discussion of the "female athlete triad" (eating disorders, irregular menses, and osteoporosis), which can be common in young female gymnasts.

2. The physical examination should be systematic and include inspection, ROM, palpation, neuro (strength, sensation, reflexes), and special tests specific to a knee examination (e.g., Lachman's, Anterior/Poster Drawer, Varus/Valgus stress, McMurray's test, Patella apprehension). A proper functional lower extremity and spine neuromuscular evaluation is essential in the comprehensive evaluation.

3. Differential diagnosis: Medial femoral condylar stress fracture, osteochondritis dissecans, medial meniscal tear, patellofemoral pain, medial plica syndrome.

4. Tests: X-rays (appropriate given the weight-bearing demands of gymnastics and potential risk of stress fracture) and MRI (could wait on MRI and start a treatment program with reassessment in 1–2 weeks or consider obtaining an MRI given the concern for a stress fracture and impact of upcoming competition).

5. Treatment includes decreased weight-bearing with use of crutches if significant pain, alternative cardiovascular training (i.e., swimming), physical therapy to improve flexibility and strength. Allow non-weight-bearing exercises with a focus on upper body and core.

6. Important points:
   a. The parents, athlete, and coach, as appropriate, should be counseled regarding the diagnosis and risks/benefits of continuing to train on the injured leg.
   b. The physician should express empathy toward the patient regarding the pressures placed on athletes and importance of the upcoming competition, discuss reasonable expectations after a stress fracture, and reassure her that she should be able to return to sport following a period of rest and rehabilitation.

7. A stress fracture is a common overuse injury that comes from repeated stress onto bone after a sudden change or increase in activity. The repetitive stress can increase bone breakdown, which can weaken the bone and make it at risk of developing small fractures that often are not seen on plain x-ray.

BIBLIOGRAPHY

De Souza MJ, Nattiv A, Joy E, et al. 2014 Female Athlete Triad Coalition consensus statement on treatment and return to play of the female athlete triad: 1st International Conference held in San Francisco, CA, May 2012, and 2nd International Conference held in Indianapolis, IN, May 2013. *Clin J Sport Med.* March 2014;24(2):96–119. https://doi.org/10.1136/bjsports-2013-093218

Mountjoy M, Sundgot-Borgen JK, Burke LM, et al. IOC consensus statement on relative energy deficiency in sport (RED-S): 2018 update. *Br J Sports Med.* June 2018;52(11):687–697. https://doi.org/10.1136/bjsports-2018-099193

Overlin AJ, Chima B, Erickson S. Update on artistic gymnastics. *Curr Sports Med Rep.* September–October 2011;10(5):304. https://doi.org/10.1249/JSR.0b013e31822dc3b2

An 18-year-old male football player presents with 1 day of right knee pain after being struck on the outside of his knee. Past medical history is unremarkable.

Questions

1. What key elements do you want to know from his history?

2. What is critical to do on physical exam?

He was attempting to cut when he was hit on the outside of the knee. He felt a popping sensation, swelling, and had difficulty weight-bearing on the leg. Examination reveals normal alignment, an effusion, and a 5-degree extension lag. He is neurovascularly intact. He has significant guarding with instability testing.

3. What is the differential diagnosis?

4. What diagnostic testing, if any, is indicated, and why?

X-rays of the right knee are normal. MRI of the knee reveals an anterior cruciate ligament (ACL) tear and meniscal tear.

5. What interventions would you recommend?

The patient got the MRI before it was authorized by insurance and is upset that he got "stuck" with the bill.

6. How do you respond? How might care be facilitated? Did the patient's presentation warrant advanced imaging?

He is worried about playing in college and developing further injury.

7. How would you counsel him?

Answers

1. The history should include a comprehensive but focused evaluation of an acute traumatic injury in the athlete. In football, one should be concerned about fractures and ligament injuries. Specific questions should include mechanism of injury (e.g., contact vs non-contact, deceleration, cutting, twisting), self-reported instability (e.g., buckling, give-way), locking and/or swelling. The history should include characterizing pain, localization of the pain, provocative and alleviating maneuvers, constitutional symptoms, and any prior injury to the knee.

2. The physical examination should be systematic and include inspection, ROM, palpation, neuro (strength, sensation, reflexes), and special tests specific for a knee examination (e.g., Lachman's, anterior/posterior Drawer, Varus/Valgus stress, McMurray's test, Patella apprehension). A proper functional lower extremity is essential in the comprehensive evaluation, though difficult in this case.

3. Differential diagnosis: ACL sprain, medial collateral ligament (MCL) sprain, meniscus tear, tibial plateau fracture.

4. Tests
   a. X-rays (appropriate given the trauma to the knee and concern for fracture)
   b. MRI (could wait on MRI and start a treatment program with reassessment in 1 to 2 weeks OR consider obtaining an MRI given the concern for significant ligament, meniscal, or bone injury).

5. Treatment includes decreased weight-bearing with use of crutches, physical therapy for modalities and to improve flexibility and strength, bracing for protection, and consideration of orthopedic referral.

6. Important points:
   a. The physician should acknowledge the patient being upset about this situation. Offer to advocate for the patient and talk to the patient's insurance about why the MRI should be covered.
   b. Factors warranting an MRI in this patient were concerns for an ACL tear, pain with weight-bearing, and knee effusion in the setting of normal knee x-rays.

7. The athlete should be counseled regarding the diagnosis of an ACL/meniscal tear, nonoperative versus operative treatment, probability of returning to the same level of play, and risk of arthritis given the type of injury.

BIBLIOGRAPHY

Montalvo AM, Schneider DK, Webster KE, et al. Anterior cruciate ligament injury risk in sport: a systematic review and meta-analysis of injury incidence by sex and sport classification. *J Athl Train*. May 2019;54(5):472–482. https://doi.org/10.4085/1062-6050-407-16

Reid D, Leigh W, Wilkins S, et al. A 10-year retrospective review of functional outcomes of adolescent anterior cruciate ligament reconstruction. *J Pediatr Orthop*. July 9, 2015;37(2):133–137. https://doi.org/10.1097/BPO.0000000000000594

Salzler M, Nwachukwu BU, Rosas S, et al. State-of-the-art anterior cruciate ligament tears: a primer for primary care physicians. *Phys Sportsmed*. May 2015;43(2):169–177. https://doi.org/10.1080/00913847.2015.1016865

A 17-year old high school high jumper presents with 2 days of left knee pain and swelling. Past medical history is unremarkable.

Questions

1. What key elements do you want to know from his history?

2. What is critical to do on physical exam?

He was attempting to jump at practice when he felt a sudden pop in his knee and fell to the ground. He reported being in excruciating pain until he straightened his knee out and the pain improved. He noted acute swelling. He denies pain with weight-bearing. Examination reveals moderate knee effusion and tenderness along the medial patellar border. He is neurovascularly intact. He has significant guarding with passive movement of his patella laterally.

3. What is the differential diagnosis?

4. What diagnostic testing, if any, is indicated, and why?

X-rays of the right knee are normal. MRI is unavailable. You diagnose the athlete with a patellar dislocation.

5. What interventions would you recommend?

The patient is requesting an MRI of his knee.

6. How do you address his request for imaging?

The patient's coach is pressuring him to return to practice as soon as possible for an event in 2 weeks.

7. How would you counsel him and resolve this conflict?

Answers

1. The history should include a comprehensive but focused evaluation of a knee injury in the athlete. The history should include localization of the pain, provocative and alleviating maneuvers, sensation of knee instability, mechanical locking symptoms, and any prior injury to the knee.

2. The physical examination should be systematic and include inspection, ROM, palpation, neuro (strength, sensation, reflexes), and special tests specific for a knee examination (e.g., Lachman's, anterior/posterior Drawer, Varus/ Valgus stress, McMurray's test, Patella apprehension). A proper functional lower extremity exam is essential in the comprehensive evaluation, including weight-bearing/walking and jumping/squatting.

3. Differential diagnosis: Patellar dislocation, ACL tear, patellar tendonitis/tear, meniscal tear, avulsion fracture, osteochondral defect.

4. Tests:
   a. X-rays (appropriate given the trauma to the knee and concern for fracture)
   b. MRI (could wait on MRI and start a treatment program with reassessment in 34 weeks or consider obtaining an MRI given the concern for significant ligament or meniscal injury, osteochondral defect).

5. Treatment includes rest, ice/heat, compression, elevation, physical therapy for modalities and to improve strength and ROM, and knee bracing for patellar stabilization.

6. Important points:
   a. The physician should express understanding about the patient's concerns, goals and natural history of patellar dislocations, including nonoperative and operative treatment.
   b. The physician should discuss indications for an MRI (assessing for osteochondral defect, injury to the medial retinaculum/MCFL).

7. The athlete, parents, coach, and athletic trainer should be counseled on the risks/benefits of returning to sport with his injury and the physician should empathize with the athlete and the pressures placed on him.

BIBLIOGRAPHY

Longo UG, Ciuffreda M, Locher J, et al. Treatment of primary acute patellar dislocation: systematic review and quantitative synthesis of the literature. *Clin J Sport Med.* 2017;27(6):511–523. https://doi.org/10.1097/JSM.0000000000000410

Smith TO, Donell S, Song F, et al. Surgical versus non-surgical interventions for treating patellar dislocation. *Cochrane Database Syst Rev.* 2015;(2):CD008106. Published 2015 Feb 26. https://doi.org/10.1002/14651858.CD008106.pub3

CASE 7

A healthy 32-year-old female tennis player presents to your sports medicine clinic with a chief complaint of right hip pain.

Questions

1. What more do you want to know about the patient's history, comorbidities, and social situation? Please tell me why you are asking for these specifics.

2. How would you go about performing a physical exam on this patient? Why are these maneuvers/exam components important?

Pain started 3 weeks ago while playing tennis. She was shuffling to her right when she noticed the pain. Pain is in the groin and lateral hip with pain in the anterior thigh. Pain is a constant dull ache with intermittent sharp pains with activity. It has worsened with time as she has continued to play tennis. Pain is worsened with activity such as walking, pivoting/turning, or playing tennis, and improved with rest. She denies numbness, tingling, and weakness. There is no popping or locking of the hip, but she does feel unstable at times. She has no history of stress fractures or bone density problems. She has no dietary restrictions. Age of menarche is 13, with normal menses.

On physical exam, she has an antalgic gait. There is tenderness to palpation of anterior hip and minimal tenderness over lateral hip. She has a normal neurological exam. Her lumbar spine and knee ROM is normal and pain-free. Passive hip ROM on the left is normal and pain-free. On the right, she has pain with hip flexion, internal rotation, and restricted internal rotation range. She has positive FADIR (flexion, adduction, internal rotation) and hip scour. Stinchfield (resisted straight leg raise) is positive. Patrick's/FABER (flexion, abduction, external rotation) is negative and provides some relief of pain. Heel strike and fulcrum test are negative. Hop test is painful on the right. She demonstrates weakness of hip abductors with single-leg squat.

3. What is the differential diagnosis for this patient? Tell me the most likely diagnosis and why.

4. What diagnostic test or tests would you order and why?

X-rays of the right hip demonstrate small cam deformity and minimal degenerative changes. Diagnostic hip injection is positive in that her pain resolves. Magnetic resonance (MR) arthrogram demonstrates small superior acetabular labral tear and minimal degenerative changes of the right hip.

5. Outline the treatment plan. Please tell me the initial treatment and next steps if that fails.

You order an MR arthrogram of the hip but the patient's insurance denies the study.

6. How might you proceed in this case?

The patient's husband is concerned that physical therapy is just a waste of time and money and asks why you are not just referring her to the surgeon first.

7. How would you counsel them?

Answers

1. History should include pain characteristics, location, severity, onset/duration/ progression, and aggravating/alleviating factors. The location of pain and presence of radiating pain is important to help to form a differential diagnosis (groin pain vs. trochanteric vs. radicular). You should ask about current activity level and any prior hip injuries. Review of systems should include numbness/tingling (nerve injury or lumbar radicular pain), weakness, and popping/locking/instability (mechanical symptoms which may stem from a labral injury). You should find determine if there is a history of stress fractures and bone density problems, and ask about dietary restrictions and menstrual history (risk for stress fractures, female athlete triad). Social history, including alcohol use (risk factor for avascular necrosis [AVN]), is also important.

2. The physical exam for hip pain includes general appearance, gait, muscle strength, neurological exam including reflexes and sensation in lower extremities, and exam of the lumbar spine and hip. Spine and hip exam includes ROM, palpation of lumbar spine and hip girdle, and special tests including FABER/Patrick's, FADIR, hip scour, heel strike/hop/fulcrum (stress fracture tests). These tests help to localize the source of pain as being intra-articular or extra-articular and helps to rule in/out referred pain from the lumbar spine. You can also include functional evaluation of hip abductor strength through single-leg stance and single-leg squat.

3. The differential diagnosis includes hip impingement, hip osteoarthritis, labral tear, femoral stress fracture, AVN, lumbar radiculitis, or femoral neuropathy. Primary hip joint pathology is the most likely pain generator given the location of her pain and reproduction with FADIR and hip scour maneuvers.

4. Hip x-ray first (including AP and lateral views) to evaluate for early osteoarthritis or femoroacetabular impingement (FAI) morphology. A diagnostic hip injection with lidocaine ± steroid can be done to confirm an intra-articular source of pain. An MR arthrogram of the hip can be done to evaluate for a labral tear and rule out other pathology such as a stress fracture.

5. Treatment options include analgesic medications as needed for pain (acetaminophen, nonsteroidal anti-inflammatory drugs [NSAIDs]), activity modification to avoid aggravating activities, and physical therapy to address possible biomechanical deficits and teach appropriate movements. Intra-articular steroid injection can be utilized if other treatments fail, and ultimately the patient can be referred to an orthopedic surgeon for arthroscopic surgery if conservative measures fail to relieve pain and/or allow return to activity.

6. You can proceed with conservative management without advanced imaging and provide reassurance to the patient that it is safe to do so. Alternatively, you could call the patient's insurance company to perform a peer-to-peer review with a physician reviewer. You can explain your concerns and how

the study would change your management plan, including the potential for interventions or surgery and lack of diagnosis based on x-rays.

7. First, you want to reassure them that you understand the concerns and that there is no harm done in waiting for surgery. Discuss that physical therapy is the appropriate first-line treatment and can provide good resolution of symptoms and allow for a return to sport and desired activities without surgery, which carries higher risks and does not guarantee a successful outcome. Physical therapy can address the biomechanical issues and weaknesses that contributed to injury, and will be helpful in the long run even if she does proceed to surgery, in which case it can be thought of "prehabilitation."

BIBLIOGRAPHY

Bruckner P, Khan K, Kemp J, et al. Hip pain. In: Brukner P, Clarsen B, Cook J, et al., eds. *Brukner & Khan's Clinical Sports Medicine.* 5th ed. McGraw-Hill Australia; 2017:593–628.

Groh MM, Herrera J. A comprehensive review of hip labral tears. *Curr Rev Musculoskelet Med.* 2009;2(2):105–117. https://doi.org/10.1007/s12178-009-9052-9

Prather H, Cheng A. Diagnosis and treatment of hip girdle pain in the athlete. *PM&R.* 2016;8:S45–S60. https://doi.org/10.1016/j.pmrj.2015.12.009

CASE 8

A healthy 15-year-old male high school cross country athlete presents to your sports medicine clinic with a chief complaint of left leg pain.

Questions

1. What more do you want to know about the patient's history, comorbidities, and social situation? Please tell me why you are asking for these specifics.

2. How would you go about performing a physical exam on this patient? Why are these maneuvers/exam components important?

Pain is in the anteromedial shin along the posteromedial tibia. It started 3 weeks ago as he started increasing the distances he was running in cross country practices with his school team and switched to running on pavement rather than the track. Pain is absent at rest. With activity, pain is located anteriorly in the right shin and is rated 8/10. Initially, pain would subside as he continued running, but now it persists. He has had to stop running due to the pain. Pain has improved some since he stopped running in the last few days. Pain worsens with walking and running and is improved with rest. He denies numbness, tingling, weakness, and lower extremity swelling.

On exam, he has symmetric 2+ dorsalis pedis and posterior tibial pulses. Strength and sensation are normal in the lower extremities. He has increased pronation with ambulation. There is diffuse tenderness to palpation along the middle third of the posteromedial tibial border. He has reduced dorsiflexion ROM with the knee flexed. His pain is reproduced with the tuning fork test.

3. What is the differential diagnosis for this patient? Tell me the most likely diagnosis and why.

4. What diagnostic test or tests would you order and why?

X-ray of the leg is negative. MRI demonstrates periosteal edema on T2-weighted images along the middle third of the posteromedial tibial border. You diagnose medial tibial stress syndrome (MTSS). CT scan is unavailable.

5. Outline the treatment plan. Please tell me the initial treatment and next steps if that fails.

He has an important cross country meet in a week and wants to compete.

6. What factors would you incorporate in addressing this ethical dilemma?

He asks about "shin splints" and asks how this is different.

7. How do you explain this to the person in lay terms?

Answers

1. History should include pain characteristics, location, severity, onset/duration, and aggravating/alleviating factors. For runners it is important to ask about precipitating factors, such as a change in training or footwear, as this can hint toward an etiology of pain and help with determining treatment. If there is pain with weight-bearing or walking, you may think more about a stress injury. You should ask if he has any prior leg injuries or prior bone stress injuries. Review of systems should include weakness, numbness/tingling, cramping, and swelling to evaluate for neurologic or vascular etiologies for his symptoms.

2. Physical exam should include a lower extremity neuromuscular exam and a more focused exam of the lower extremities including alignment, foot structure, ankle/foot alignment with ambulation, and ankle ROM with knee flexed and extended to assess for both gastrocnemius and soleus tightness. You should palpate along the anterior and medial portions of the tibia and along the fibula to evaluate for areas of possible stress injury. A tuning fork test can also be done as a test for stress fracture. You should evaluate distal pulses to rule out vascular cause of exertional leg pain. Hip ROM should also be evaluated as increased hip external rotation is a risk factor for MTSS.

3. Differential diagnosis: MTSS (shin splints), tibial stress fracture, chronic exertional compartment syndrome, muscle strain, vascular compression (usually popliteal), metabolic bone disease, bony tumor (osteosarcoma, osteoid osteoma), lumbar radicular pain.

4. X-rays can be done to evaluate for obvious stress fracture but will often be negative even in the setting of fracture. Bone scans are not as specific as MRI, which is the test of choice that can differentiate MTSS and stress fracture and help grade stress fractures, which can direct treatment and provide prognostic information. Other tools in evaluation of exertional leg pain include compartment pressure testing (pre- and post-exertion), ankle brachial index (ABI), MR angiogram, and EMG/NCS. CT is not indicated and should be avoided due to the radiation exposure, especially in young patients.

5. Treatment includes rest from aggravating activities and treating the underlying pathology. Ice and analgesics (acetaminophen, NSAIDs) can be used. The athlete should be allowed to cross-train with pain-free activities such as swimming or cycling to maintain cardiovascular fitness. Immobilization and protected weight-bearing in knee-high walking boot or pneumatic stirrup leg brace may be required. For excessive pronation, appropriate footwear and orthotics that include cushion and medial arch support are indicated. A course of physical therapy to address stretching and strengthening is recommended. When pain free, he can pursue a gradual return to sport.

6. It is important to empathize with him but advise him of the risks involved if he were to continue to run. There is the possibility that if he continues to run, he

could develop a stress fracture. That would then be more difficult to manage, potentially requiring a period of non-weight-bearing and strict avoidance of activity. There is even the possibility that it would require surgery if he had a higher risk anterior tibial fracture. The appropriate treatment is rest and addressing necessary biomechanical issues to prevent recurrence and progression. He should then have a quicker and more successful return to sport with a lower likelihood of future injuries.

7. This condition, MTSS, is what some people refer to as "shin splints." However, sometimes the term "shin splints" is used to describe any lower leg pain that occurs with exercise, not just MTSS.

The medical term that we use provides a more accurate description of the problem, which is stress along the inside (medial) portion of the shin bone (tibia). The muscles pull along the attachment on the bone and that produces pain as the bone gets inflamed (stress reaction). It is important that the athlete knows their diagnosis and the risks associated so they can make informed decisions. It is possible they may also be able to help teammates in the future who have the same problem.

BIBLIOGRAPHY

Bruckner P, Khan K, Hutchison M, et al. Leg pain. In: Brukner P, Clarsen B, Cook J, et al., eds. *Brukner & Khan's Clinical Sports Medicine.* 5th ed. McGraw-Hill Australia; 2017:593–628.

Johnson S. Exertional leg pain in runners. In: Harrast M. *Clinical Care of the Runner.* 1st ed. Elsevier; 2020:215–229. https://doi.org/10.1016/B978-0-323-67949-7.00019-7

Rajasekaran S, Finnoff JT. Exertional leg pain. *Phys Med Rehabil Clin N Am.* 2016;27:91–119. https://doi.org/10.1016/j.pmr.2015.08.012

A 45-year-old male runner presents to your sports medicine clinic with chief complaint of right posterior ankle pain.

Questions

1. What more do you want to know about the patient's history, co-morbidities, and social situation? Please tell me why you are asking for these specifics.

2. How would you go about performing a physical exam on this patient? Why are these maneuvers/exam components important?

His pain started gradually a month ago with running and has increased with time. He had increased his running volume around the time of onset. He has continued to run but is running shorter distances as pain increases with running. He has noticed swelling of the Achilles tendon. He had also taken a course of ciprofloxacin a couple months ago.

On exam, he is overweight with body mass index (BMI) of 29. He has tenderness to palpation over a focal thickening of the Achilles tendon about 3 cm proximal to its insertion on the calcaneus. Ankle ROM is full. When walking he has pronation of the ankle. He has a normal neurologic exam including strength although resisted plantarflexion on the affected right side is painful.

3. What is the differential diagnosis for this patient? Tell me the most likely diagnosis and why.

4. What diagnostic test or tests would you order and why?

X-rays of the right ankle are normal. Ultrasound demonstrates focal thickening of the mid-portion of the Achilles tendon consistent with Achilles tendinopathy. MRI is not available.

5. Outline the treatment plan. Please tell me initial treatment and next steps if that fails.

The patient states that he does not have the time to attend physical therapy due to his busy work schedule which also involves a lot of travel.

6. How would you help to facilitate his physical therapy?

The patient would like you to explain the recommended exercise program to him so he can do it on his own at home.

7. How would you explain eccentric exercises to the patient and how would you recommend he perform these exercises for this problem?

Answers

1. History should include pain location (Achilles insertion, mid-portion, muscle), onset/progression, and quality. You should ask if there was a specific injury including feeling or hearing a pop and any bruising (possible Achilles rupture or gastrocnemius strain). If there is any swelling or thickening of the tendon this can lead you to a diagnosis of tendinopathy or bursitis. You should ask about any changes in training (terrain, speed, volume), exercise, or footwear around the time of symptom onset. What are the aggravating and alleviating factors? History of prior ankle injuries should be included as this can increase risk of further injuries or ankle arthritis. Review of systems to include recent antibiotic use (fluoroquinolones can increase risk of Achilles rupture), numbness/tingling, or weakness (lumbar radiculopathy in an S1 distribution could be a cause of posterior ankle pain).

2. Physical exam should include BMI. A lower extremity neurologic exam should be included to rule out radiculopathy. CV exam of distal pulses to rule out vascular etiology. Include inspection of lower extremity alignment, foot structure including arch, and ankle/foot alignment with ambulation for biomechanical contributors to his symptoms. Palpate along the Achilles tendon to determine location of pain (mid-portion or insertion) and evaluate for focal thickening of the tendon which is seen in tendinopathy. As the ankle is moved into plantarflexion/dorsiflexion you can also palpate for crepitus of the tendon suggestive of tendinopathy and to determine if the site of pain moves in relation to the malleoli (suggestive of tendon pathology) and if it improves with maximum dorsiflexion (Royal London Hospital test for Achilles tendinopathy). Evaluate ROM of the ankle and foot including with knee flexed and extended to assess for both gastrocnemius and soleus tightness. Thompson test can rule out Achilles tendon rupture.

3. Differential diagnosis: Achilles tendinopathy (mid-portion or insertional), retrocalcaneal bursitis, Haglund's syndrome, gastrocnemius strain, calcaneus stress fracture, Achilles rupture, peroneal tendinopathy, lumbar radicular pain, osteomyelitis, bony tumor, flexor hallucis longus or tibialis posterior tendinopathy, os trigonum syndrome, posterior impingement syndrome.

4. Tests: X-rays can be done to evaluate for bony abnormality such as a Haglund deformity which can contribute to Achilles pain. Ultrasound can be done to further evaluate the structure of the Achilles tendon and evaluate for tendinopathy. MRI is an alternative option and can also be used when there is concern for a calcaneal stress fracture. CT scan is generally not indicated.

5. Treatment generally begins with rest from aggravating activities and treating the underlying pathology. For pain management, ice and analgesics (acetaminophen, NSAIDs) can be used. A heel lift can help to reduce load on the Achilles to provide symptomatic relief. Orthotics are used to correct biomechanical problems. Immobilization and protected weight-bearing in a walking

boot is used only in severe cases. A course of physical therapy to address stretching and strengthening is recommended; eccentric strengthening and heavy slow resistance training have been shown to be equivalent and effective. For recalcitrant cases, extracorporeal shockwave therapy (ESWT), nitric oxide via topical glyceryl trinitrate (GTN) patches, and procedures can be pursued. Peritendinous corticosteroid injections can be performed with caution as there is possible increased risk of tendon rupture with these injections. Needle tenotomy and injections of autologous blood or platelet rich plasma (PRP) are also options.

6. When patients report inability to attend physical therapy due to schedule or other concerns, it may be best to provide the patient a home exercise program if feasible. Other options are to encourage the patient to attend even one or two visits of physical therapy to have assessment with the therapist and to be taught a home exercise program.

7. Explain that eccentric exercises involve exercising the muscle while elongating the muscle/tendon unit. For the Achilles, the eccentric program involves rising up onto toes (ankle plantarflexion) on a stair while standing on both legs then lowering down slowly on the affected side until the heel is lower than the stair (dorsiflexed). It is important not to put too much load on the affected side during the concentric phase when the muscle is being shortened. In the setting of insertional tendinopathy this exercise would be modified to avoid dorsiflexion so it is done on a flat surface rather than edge of a stair.

BIBLIOGRAPHY

Bruckner P, Khan K, Cook J, et al. Pain in the Achilles region. In: Brukner P, Clarsen B, Cook J, et al., eds. *Brukner & Khan's clinical sports medicine.* 5th ed. McGraw-Hill Australia; 2017:865–892.

Deakins-Roche M, Fredericson M, Kraus E. Ankle and foot injuries in runners. In: Harrast M, ed. *Clinical care of the runner.* 1st ed. Elsevier; 2020:231–245.

Maffuli N, Longo UG, Kadakia A, et al. Achilles tendinopathy. *Foot Ankle Surg.* 2020;26:240–249. https://doi.org/10.1016/j.fas.2019.03.009

16 Stroke Rehabilitation

Benjamin J. Friedman, Deena Hassaballa, and Richard L. Harvey

A 70-year-old male with a history of hypertension and diabetes mellitus is admitted to acute inpatient rehabilitation following a left middle cerebral artery (MCA) distribution ischemic stroke. He has a right hemiparesis, aphasia, and moderate dysphagia. In the first week of his rehabilitation stay (10 days post-stroke), staff is noting that the patient is easily frustrated, demonstrating more apathy and poor effort, and "not the same as he was when he got here last week." His nurse asked that you evaluate him.

Questions

1. What would you like to know about history/review of systems (ROS) and physical exam (PE) to evaluate the staff's concerns? Please tell me why you are asking for these specifics.

His examination is similar to that on admission 10 days ago: a moderate mixed aphasia (nonfluent with mild comprehension deficits), a right hemiparesis with early signs of hypertonia in the upper extremity (UE), no fevers or signs of infection, and a flat affect. ROS includes decreased appetite, sadness, and frustration with his communication changes, and he denies suicidal ideation. No recent medication changes have been made.

2. What screening tools will help establish a diagnosis of post-stroke depression (PSD)?

The examination and screening tools suggest mild-moderate depressive symptoms.

3. Please outline the treatment plan. Please tell me the initial treatment and next steps if that fails.

The patient's daughter shared that he was widowed 2 years ago, and "He had handled the loss well, but I have never seen him like this." She wants to know what risk factors are associated with PSD, and what his prognosis might be.

4. What are the risk factors for PSD?

5. What are the physical problems associated with PSD?

His daughter then states, "Ever since mom passed, dad was always saying he will not take antidepressants because of what they did to her." She thinks, based on the information you had explained earlier, that he should take them, but she says "I can't force him," and asks you to "talk him into it."

6. How do you approach this situation and to resolve the potential conflict?

Answers

1. Ask about prior history of depression or anxiety as it has been shown to be an increased risk factor for PSD. Determine the severity of his functional deficits—lower Barthel scores have also been associated with increased depression. Inquire if any recent event happened since he had arrived for rehabilitation—for example, fall or head trauma. Ask additional questions to help narrow down the differential of causes that can be contributing to his symptoms. Does he have anhedonia or appetite changes (signs of depression)? What is the severity of his aphasia? Are there reversible conditions that can be causing a delirium (e.g., infections, recent medication changes, constipation, urinary retention)? Does he have insomnia or a sleep disturbance? Are there any pain complaints that may be impacting sleep, mood, and participation in therapy?

2. Question the patient directly about depression (multiple screening tools available: Patient Health Questionnaire-2 [PHQ-2], PHQ-9, Beck Depression Inventory-II [BDI-II], Geriatric Depression Scale [GDS], Stroke Aphasic Depression Questionnaire-Hospital Version [SADQ-H]). PSD is very common, underdiagnosed, and can impact a patient's rehabilitation and recovery. This is especially true in stroke patients with aphasia as recent studies have shown that due to their communication deficits, they are at a higher risk of not being screened or diagnosed. Suicide screening is necessary and should be incorporated into all practices.

3. Initially, offer antidepressants and possibly a stimulant as well as psychotherapy. After that, consider a stimulant medication if the patient is having significant apathy or lethargy. There is no evidence that one selective serotonin reuptake inhibitor (SSRI) is more efficacious than another, and they have been generally well tolerated and are not associated with an increased risk in mortality. Most studies have tested sertraline and citalopram. The choice of medication requires the physiatrist to balance the benefits versus the side effects and adjust dose as needed. Review the benefits of exercise for depression and encourage participation with therapy. Note that programs of 4 weeks duration have been studied to show a complementary benefit for PSD. Provide education, counseling, and support about the stroke, and provide the patient and their family the opportunity to speak about the impact of the illness on their lives. Consider psychiatric evaluation if mood disorder is causing persistent distress or worsening disability. Explain that monitoring of symptoms and responses to treatment will be continued while in rehab and upon discharge.

4. Prior psychiatric illness, Asevere stroke and disability, and cognitive impairment have a high association with PSD.

5. Incontinence, impaired mobility, sleep apnea, pain/discomfort, cognitive impairment, disability, and stroke severity (high modified Rankin scale and

NIHSS scores). Less strongly associated are limited support, socioeconomic status, and female sex. It would be beneficial to review with the patient's family that approximately one-third of stroke patients do develop clinically significant depression at some point after the stroke. It is important to note that PSD is not related to any character weakness on the patient's part, and may result from physiological changes in the brain after stroke. Approximately 40% of patients develop symptoms within 3 months of a stroke. Many stroke patients can develop depression after discharge from the inpatient rehabilitation unit. Interestingly, most patients with major PSD appear to recover significantly better than those with minor PSD by 2 years after the stroke. As mentioned, the level of disability (low Barthel index score), inadequate social support, coping style (especially catastrophic reaction and emotionalism), and a pre-stroke history of depression are early predictors of PSD.

6. You should first explain that any competent adult has the right to refuse treatment. If the patient lacks capacity, treatment decisions would be deferred to the closest family member. That said, it is worthwhile to suggest a family meeting to explore his fears, validate his concerns, and also explain the rationale of antidepressant use. He should be reassured that he will continue to be monitored. If the patient is willing to discuss this with his family present, supportive communication techniques will be needed to assure he understands given his aphasia. If a particular medication is considered, the side effects and major risk factors of its use should be discussed.

BIBLIOGRAPHY

Ashaie SA, Hurwitz R, Cherney LR. Depression and subthreshold depression in stroke-related aphasia, archives of physical medicine and rehabilitation. *Arch Phys Med Rehabil.* 2019;100(7):1294–1299. https://doi.org/10.1016/j.apmr.2019.01.024

Feng R, Wang P, Gao C, et al. Effect of sertraline in the treatment and prevention of poststroke depression: a meta-analysis. *Medicine (Baltimore).* 2018 97(49):e13453. https://doi.org/10.1097/MD.0000000000013453

Jørgensen TS, Wium-Andersen IK, Wium-Andersen MK, et al. Incidence of depression after stroke, and associated risk factors and mortality outcomes, in a large cohort of Danish patients. *JAMA Psychiatry.* 2016;73:1032–1040. https://doi.org/10.1001/jamapsychiatry.2016.1932

Towfighi A, Ovbiagele B, El Husseini N, et al. Poststroke depression: a scientific statement for healthcare professionals from the American Heart Association/American Stroke Association. *Stroke.* 2017;48:e30–e43. https://doi.org/10.1161/STR.0000000000000113

Winstein CJ, Stein J, Arena R, et al. Guidelines for adult stroke rehabilitation and recovery: a guideline for healthcare professionals from the American Heart Association/American Stroke Association. *Stroke.* 2016;6:e98–e169. https://doi.org/10.1161/STR.0000000000000098

CASE 2

A 70-year-old male with a history of stroke, which caused left hemiparesis, is having left shoulder pain that started about 10 to 12 days post-stroke.

Questions

1. What more would you like to know to help you evaluate this patient?

2. How would you go about performing a physical exam on this patient? Why are these maneuvers/exam components important?

His examination shows a subluxation of about two finger breadths, pain with passive external rotation, abduction, and flexion, with mild hypertonia and reduced range in all directions. The left upper limb remains without voluntary movement, and there is no regional sensory or temperature changes. He denies prior trauma to the shoulder but he does share that he has had stiffness in that arm even before the stroke.

3. Discuss your differential diagnosis and what can support your reasoning?

4. Based on your differential diagnosis what would you like to do next to help confirm your diagnosis and treat the patient?

X-rays of the shoulder are negative for fracture and there are no joint space narrowing, cystic changes, or osteopenia. There is a 1.5 cm subluxation noted. Musculoskeletal ultrasound showed thickening of the coracohumeral ligament and the soft tissues of the rotator cuff. There are no tears or partial tears of the rotator cuff muscles.

5. Outline the treatment plan. Please tell me the initial treatment and next steps if that fails.

His family asks what a subluxation is and if it explains his pain.

6. How will you explain the complex relationship between subluxation and pain?

On follow-up a month post-discharge from rehab, although the patient does not appear to be in severe pain at present, his family is demanding opioids for his pain and states that last week, "the urgent care doctor gave him oxycodone."

7. How would you approach this request?

Answers

1. Obtain history on prior trauma, onset of symptoms, and associated movements that exacerbate symptoms, as well as other comorbidities. Shoulder pain is very common after stroke but there are many different potential causes. Early identification, diagnosis, and treatment of hemiplegic shoulder pain reduces the risk of developing chronic shoulder pain and it allows for better participation and potential recovery. You will want to ask about the characteristics of the shoulder pain, its exact location, severity, what makes it worse, and what makes it better.

2. Inspect for deformities of the shoulder and the elbow; evaluate for restricted motion, tenderness on palpation, instability, and in what directions or motions is pain provoked. If painful motions are noted, more specific provocative maneuvers are done to differentiate which muscles or tendons are involved. Fractures of the shoulder joint, scapula, adhesive capsulitis (frozen shoulder), and degenerative joint disease of the shoulder may all have limited motion, tenderness, and pain depending on the severity of the disease or the injury. Evaluate if there is a subluxation of the shoulder, and whether or not it can be reduced. Subluxation is common in a flaccid or hypotonic hemiplegic limb. Manual muscle testing using the medical research council grading system in all four limbs is important to determine the severity of hemiplegia as well as to identify any weakness on the non-hemiplegic side. Injuries to a joint and its associated structures, and the direction the pain occurs can narrow the diagnosis. For the glenohumeral joint, provocative tests include the apprehension test, relocation test, and anterior draw test, which would support anterior glenohumeral instability. Posterior glenohumeral instability would be tested with a posterior draw test and a jerk test. A positive sulcus sign is suggestive of multidirectional instability associated with increased laxity in the glenohumeral joint. Labral tears may also show signs of instability and pain. Rotator cuff injuries may show a painful arc on testing of range of motion and positive drop arm test will often be seen in a complete tear. Signs of impingement of the supraspinatus can be elicited with the Neer's sign, which compresses the supraspinatus tendon between the acromion and the greater tuberosity. The Hawkin's sign also demonstrates supraspinatus involvement with compression against the coracoacromial ligament. Injuries of the biceps tendon and tendonitis will have point tenderness in the bicipital groove, and provocative testing can be further done including the Yergason's and Speed's tests. Limited range may be due to spasticity or contracture, and this should be assessed using the modified Ashworth Scale or the Tardieu scale. If the patient has spasticity, examination of the shoulder range in the supine position is preferred in order to eliminate postural hypertonia. Skin sensation should be examined because of sensory loss from the stroke and to confirm that these changes do not follow a dermatomal pattern. Sensory changes can be seen with proximal humerus fractures and traction injuries to the brachial plexus or distal peripheral nerves. Complex regional pain syndrome (CRPS) may have sensory and skin color changes.

3. Subluxation is very common in stroke patients with hemiplegia; however, the association with subluxation and shoulder pain is controversial. The reason is that severe hemiplegia is strongly associated with later development of shoulder pain and subluxation is associated with hemiplegia. While managing and limiting the subluxation is part of the treatment plan, it is important to ensure that there are no other factors that can be contributing to the patient's discomfort. A thorough examination of the shoulder should be performed as well as plain x-ray imaging, shoulder ultrasound, or other radiographic methods in order to clarify the mechanical source of pain. It is important to prevent trauma to the shoulder in a patient with a severely weak upper limb. In hemiplegia, the rotator cuff sleeve is not able to maintain the humeral head in the glenoid and the scapula is downward rotated, predisposing to subluxation. Poor positioning in bed or wheelchair, lack of support when upright, or traction on the arm during transfers can cause soft tissue injury, leading to pain. Pain on passive range of motion is suggestive of rotator cuff pathology, impingement syndrome, or adhesive capsulitis. A history of diabetes mellitus can also predispose to adhesive capsulitis.

4. Early identification and managing shoulder pain in patients with hemiparesis has been shown to be beneficial, especially prior to discharge from rehabilitation. Evaluate the limb for spasticity and implement noninvasive treatments (stretching, splinting/orthosis, electrical stimulation, cold and heat modalities) prior to medications (oral vs. intramuscular). Imaging with plain film x-ray (to evaluate for fracture, osteoarthritis, and severity of subluxation) and/or musculoskeletal ultrasound prior to MRI (due to cost) or arthrogram (invasive)—to demonstrate rotator cuff pathology and fibrosis of tendons. Corticosteroid injections for decreasing inflammation in rotator cuff partial tear injuries, adhesive capsulitis, impingement syndromes, and tendinitis may allow for improvement in range of motion with therapy. These can play both a diagnostic and therapeutic role. Ideally, CRPS should be identified early in its course. Triple phase bone scanning is beneficial in the first 3 months, as x-ray changes will not demonstrate the demineralization that is needed for detection. If CRPS is suspected, a pulse of oral steroids can be beneficial; however, this is relatively contraindicated in diabetics. Sympathetic blockade of the stellate ganglion is used for sympathetically mediated CRPS type I. Nerve injury or traction neuropathy should be evaluated clinically in cases where atypical motor recovery is noted, when finger extensor contracture is seen, with segmental muscle atrophy, and delayed onset of spasticity. It can be evaluated by electromyography (EMG) to demonstrate lower motor neuron findings.

5. The earlier imaging studies were done to rule out other pathologies of the shoulder. The ultrasound findings do support a diagnosis of adhesive capsulitis. Initial treatment includes proper positioning, maintaining the arm in a functional position. To protect the hemiplegic shoulder from further injury, proper positioning and support of the limb is provided during all aspects of his care. Supporting the arm in bed with pillows and use of an arm trough or lap tray on wheelchair is critically important. If there is pain or instability during ambulation, a sling that allows the arm to remain in a functional

position may be used. It is important to provide education to caregivers and family members about the need for proper positioning, support, and correct performance of passive range of motion and stretching in order to prevent further injury. Therapy is prescribed to address restrictions on shoulder range of motion. Modalities with cold and/or heat, electrical stimulation, and acetaminophen and or nonsteroidal anti-inflammatory drugs (NSAIDS; if not contraindicated) may be used for pain control. If painful symptoms persist, intra-articular glucocorticoid injection followed by continued therapy to increase range of motion. If spasticity is a major component, then botulinum toxin injections to the pectorals and subscapularis may be indicated.

6. Discuss what a subluxation is and describe the separation of the humeral head from the glenoid fossa; however, also note that he has signs of adhesive capsulitis and review the treatment plan that was outlined earlier. In explaining subluxation, use lay terms and consider use of a diagram for illustrative purposes. Explain how unattended subluxation may lead to shoulder injury which results in pain, but the subluxation alone is not the cause of pain. For this patient, who also has adhesive capsulitis, treatment focuses on restoration of range of motion with therapy as well as limiting of inflammation and pain with analgesics, electrical stimulation, and corticosteroid injections in order to maximize participation in therapy.

7. First, confirm on exam that there are no new changes such as spasticity or signs of CRPS and if not, then discuss the patient's pain and its mechanisms. If there is concern for lack of a response to the current treatments, inquire about whether the patient and family were fully compliant with the previous treatment plan. It would also be important to screen the patient for risk factors of substance abuse. Check with patient's pharmacy and/or the state's prescription monitoring program to identify any aberrant behavior in opioid use. If you determine that opioid medications would be useful for pain control, review with the patient and the family member that an opiate use agreement would need to be signed and that there should be only a single prescribing physician to allow for safe and proper dosing. It is recommended to review with the family that the most common reason for ED visits from opioid overdose is a family member using a patient's medication.

BIBLIOGRAPHY

Kalichman L, Ratmansky M. Underlying pathology and associated factors of hemiplegic shoulder pain. *Am J Phys Med Rehabil*. 2011;90:768–780. https://doi.org/10.1097/PHM.0b013e318214e976

Suh CH, Yun SJ, Jin W, et al. Systematic review and meta-analysis of magnetic resonance imaging features for diagnosis of adhesive capsulitis of the shoulder. *Eur Radiol*. 2019;29:566–577. https://doi.org/10.1007/s00330-018-5604-y

Winstein CJ, Stein J, Arena R, et al. Guidelines for adult stroke rehabilitation and recovery: a guideline for healthcare professionals from the American Heart Association/American Stroke Association. *Stroke*. 2016;6:e98–e169. https://doi.org/10.1161/STR.0000000000000098

CASE 3

A 69-year-old man with a history of hypertension, obesity, and diabetes, whom you cared for after a right MCA stroke 5 years prior, presents to your outpatient clinic for the first time in 3 years. He lives independently and was doing well until about a month ago, when he started having pain in his left foot while walking.

Questions

1. What more do you want to know about the patient's history, comorbidities, and social situation? Please tell me why you are asking for these specifics.

2. How would you go about performing a physical exam on this patient? Why are these maneuvers/exam components important?

Your patient tells you that he lives alone in a condominium and takes care of all his personal needs. He walks with a quad cane and left ankle-foot orthosis (AFO), but he admits that he does not like the AFO and usually does not wear it unless he leaves the house. Over the last month, he has noted a deep aching and burning pain in the bottom of his foot when walking with the AFO. He would like to get a new one that is more comfortable. He denies any history of past or recent foot injury or trauma. He says he does not regularly inspect his feet, though he was advised to do so when he was diagnosed with diabetic neuropathy. He has never had a foot ulcer. He also denies any history of claudication and has never been told he has poor circulation.

Examination shows left spastic hemiplegia. Left hip flexion is 3/5, knee extension 5/5, and ankle dorsiflexion 0/5. On the plantar surface of his left foot, there is a 1.2 × 1.5 cm ulcer with surrounding callous and a clean base. No purulence or foul smell is noted. His foot shows no obvious deformity. Passive ankle range shows a 20-degree plantarflexion contracture with a spasticity angle of 10 degrees and 5 beats of clonus on fast stretch. He has absent pinprick sensation to mid-calf in both feet. Dorsalis pedis pulse is palpable in left foot, but not the posterior tibialis pulse. Capillary refill in great toe is sluggish. When standing barefoot, his ankle assumes a plantar-flexed and slightly inverted position. He can ambulate with a stiff-knee gait without the AFO, clearing his left foot with hip-hike. His initial contact is the lateral forefoot. He has genu recurvatum throughout stance phase. You note that the AFO does not fit well, and it is quite difficult to seat the heel all the way into the orthotic.

3. What is the differential diagnosis for this patient? Tell me the most likely diagnosis and why.

4. What diagnostic test or tests would you order and why?

Laboratory tests show a normal white blood cell (WBC) and C-reactive protein (CRP). Plain films show no fracture or bony abnormality in left foot. EMG was normal but nerve conduction studies (NCS) showed loss of or slowing of sensory nerve conduction bilaterally. Ankle-brachial index (ABI) and arterial duplex were normal. Wound culture grew normal skin flora.

5. Outline the treatment plan. Please tell me the initial treatment and next steps if that fails.

This patient was last seen in your clinic 3 years ago. You look in the record and you note that you had recommended he see you in a year following your last visit. Although a follow-up appointment was made, your patient tells you he felt he was doing well at that time, and he chose to cancel. You are concerned that a diabetic with an AFO should probably be followed more closely.

6. What factors would you incorporate in addressing this clinical problem?

After several changes of the total contact cast (TCC), the ulcer is fully healed. A new custom AFO is provided as previously described. The patient becomes frustrated when you emphasize that he should wear the AFO at all times during the day, including in the house. He raises his voice, telling you, "It was the AFO that caused my ulcer! If I wear it all the time I will get another and I am not going through all that casting again!"

7. Tell me in lay terms how would you resolve this conflict?

Answers

1. The physician needs to understand this patient's current functional ability, and especially his gait function. What assistive devices does he use while walking? A clear history of any recent or past injuries, falls, or foot trauma is important. A patient with diabetes may have a history of peripheral neuropathy (PN), leading to loss of sensation or neuropathic pain. The patient may have peripheral vascular disease, which may lead to claudication or, if PN is also present, may contribute to the development of a nonhealing diabetic foot ulcer. Severe PN can result in chronic microfractures with eventual joint dislocation and collapse (Charcot foot). Furthermore, diabetic foot ulcers place the patient at risk for infection and may lead to amputation. The physician should inquire about whether the patient inspects his foot regularly for injury or skin breakdown.

2. Manual muscle testing using the medical research council grading system in all four limbs is important to determine the severity of hemiplegia as well as to identify any weakness on the non-hemiplegic side. If the patient wears an AFO, its fit should be examined and its structural integrity assessed. Skin sensation should be examined in the hemiplegic leg, including vibration sensation, pinprick, and proprioception, which may be reduced in a diabetic or because of sensory loss from the stroke. With sensory loss, there is a risk for pressure ulcer with AFO use. A chronic diabetic with PN and peripheral vascular disease (PVD) may be especially at risk for a diabetic foot ulcer from a poor-fitting AFO. Therefore, careful palpation of the dorsalis pedis and posterior tibialis pulses is important. Passive and active range is assessed and assessment for any boney deformities. Any limited ankle range (e.g., an ankle plantarflexion contracture) should be measured using a goniometer. Limited range may be due to spasticity or contracture, and this should be assessed using the modified Ashworth scale or the Tardieu scale. Measuring R1 and R2 and calculating the spasticity ankle can help differentiate contracture from spasticity (although both may be present).

3. Possible causes of a painful foot when walking with an AFO include foot fracture (including Charcot foot), poor orthotic fit, ankle contracture, pressure ulcer on foot, painful diabetic neuropathy or diabetic foot ulcer, or claudication.

4. In the presence of a foot ulcer and sensory loss, EMG with NCS of both lower limbs is appropriate. With absent pedal pulses, slow capillary refill, or a foot ulcer, it is important to obtain ABI and arterial duplex scan to assess for peripheral vascular disease. Plain x-rays including anteroposterior (AP), lateral, and oblique views of the foot should be obtained. A complete blood count (CBC), glycol-hemoglobin, erythrocyte sedimentation rate (ESR), CRP, and blood cultures should be collected. If consistent with infection, an MRI of the foot should be performed to assess for underlying osteomyelitis.

5. A TCC is recommended first to allow healing of the diabetic foot ulcer. The TCC is changed every 2 weeks until the ulcer heals. Once healed, a new AFO is custom-molded, including a heel built up to account for the 20-degree plantarflexion contracture. A lift incorporated into the right shoe may be needed as well. If spasticity remains an issue, local injection of botulinum toxin into plantar flexors and ankle invertors may help. The patient needs thorough education on daily foot inspection and to be provided with a mirror with an extended handle to facilitate full skin inspection. He is also instructed to only walk with the AFO on his foot.

6. If your practice has a clinical association with an orthotics center, you could discuss with the manager there about putting together a quality improvement project to closely follow diabetic patients from your practice who are issued orthotics. In the case described a task force was gathered from both organizations. After several meetings, the team decides to screen all diabetics for neuropathy at the time of first orthotic fitting using a 128-Hz tuning fork, assessing for a stocking-glove distribution loss of vibratory sensation. Anyone screening positive will be contacted every 6 months by an orthotist to inquire about orthotic fit and skin integrity. Any patient with concerns will be asked to come into the clinic for an assessment. The team chooses to measure the rate of referrals who screen into the program, the rate of program participants who are asked to come to the clinic, the rate of early foot ulcers identified, and the frequency of orthotic modifications made as part of the program. The team plans to meet every 6 months to review the data.

7. "I agree that it does sound odd for me to ask you to wear a brace when your ulcer happened while wearing the previous brace. We did make a new one for you and this one fits much better, so your risk of another ulcer is much less. Wearing the brace will keep your foot in a good position while walking and will actually protect your skin. But if you walk without the brace, I worry that your forefoot may experience a lot of pressure and break down again. It will be very important for you to inspect your foot daily for injury as we have discussed before. If wearing the brace all day is something you are not fully comfortable with, we could talk about surgical options to correct your ankle position. This does not eliminate your risk of skin breakdown, and it carries its own risks, but it is an option that may allow at least some walking at home without the brace."

BIBLIOGRAPHY

Ahmed S, Barwick A, Butterworth, et al. Footwear and insole design features that reduce neuropathic plantar foot ulcer risk in people with diabetes: a systematic literature review. *J Foot Ankle Res*. 2020;13:30. https://doi.org/10.1186/s13047-020-00400-4

Appasamy M, De Witt ME, Patel N, et al. Treatment strategies for genu recruvatum in adult patients with hemiparesis: a case series. *PM&R*. 2015;7:105–112. https://doi.org/10.1016/j.pmrj.2014.10.015

Chakraborty PP, Ray S, Biswas D, et al. A comparative study between total contact cast and pressure-relieving ankle foot orthosis in diabetic neuropathic foot ulcers. *J Diabetes Sci Tech*. 2015;9(2):302–308. https://doi.org/10.1177/1932296814560788

Fatone S, Malas BS. Orthotic management in stroke. In Stein J, Harvey RL, Winstein CJ, et al, eds. *Stroke Recovery and Rehabilitation*. 2nd ed. Demos Medical Publishing; 2015:589–608.

Shahabi S, Shabaninejad H, Kamali M, et al. The effects of ankle-foot orthoses on walking speed in patients with stroke: a systematic review and meta-analysis of randomized controlled trials. *Clin Rehabil*. 2020;34(2):145–159. https://doi.org/10.1177/0269215519887784

CASE 4

A 38-year-old female with a medical history of left basal ganglia hemorrhage 12 months prior had a recent fall at home associated with decrease in function and rehospitalization. She has been admitted to your acute inpatient rehabilitation service. Her participation in therapy has been limited by pain.

Questions

1. What more do you want to know about the patient's history, comorbidities, and social situation? Please tell me why you are asking for these specifics.

2. How would you go about performing a physical exam on this patient? Why are these maneuvers/exam components important?

She had an excellent return of function after her stroke and returned to part-time work as a school bus driver. The patient reports she has been having burning pain or numbness in her right arm that has gotten progressively worse. This pain started 6 months ago. It is not a constant pain but will usually wax and wane in intensity. She reports that cold temperatures make the pain worse. She denies swelling of the extremity, trauma, or weakness. She has tried acetaminophen and ibuprofen, but they do not help. She read on a stroke blog that marijuana helps, so she has been self-medicating. She lives in a state where medical marijuana use is legal, but she is too embarrassed to ask her doctors about it. On exam, the patient is awake, alert, oriented to person, place, and time; her general appearance shows a calm individual supine in bed with no grimacing noted at rest. Inspection of the skin in bilateral arm and legs is negative for erythema or swelling; light palpation along her right arm elicits slight grimacing. She has hyperalgesia with light pinprick to the right forearm and right hand. Light touch elicits allodynia in the right hand. Deep tendon reflexes are hyporeflexic throughout; sensation to light touch is intact and symmetric otherwise; muscle strength testing seems at 5/5 but quite limited by pain; cold temperature elicits significant grimacing compared to warm temperatures; two-point discrimination impaired.

3. What is the differential diagnosis for this patient? Tell me the most likely diagnosis and why.

4. What diagnostic test or tests would you order and why?

Her lab work shows no abnormalities on the complete metabolic panel (CMP), CBC, vitamin labs, and thyroid panel. X-rays of the upper and lower limb are negative. MRI and bone scan are not available at your rehabilitation center. NCS and EMG were not fully completed due to poor tolerance from the pain.

5. Outline the treatment plan. Please tell me the initial treatment and next steps if that fails.

The patient started the recommended medication duloxetine. She felt it helped her pain, but her mother warned her that it was an antidepressant and said that she should try a more natural treatment option. The patient returns to you and tells you that her friends let her try cannabis/marijuana again and she felt it helped her pain significantly. She wants you to fill out a form for medical marijuana and explains that her job as a school bus driver will not be an issue while she is on treatment.

6. What factors would you incorporate in addressing this ethical dilemma?

After another 6 months, the patient returns to your clinic in a frustrated mood and states that her pain is not completely gone and that she was under the impression the treatment for this would eradicate her pain altogether. She feels that her stroke and weakness were enough to handle but that her pain is interfering with her ability to function even more. She wants to know more about her diagnosis and treatment options.

7. Tell me in lay terms about how you would respond to her concerns.

Answers

1. It is important to obtain a full history of her pain and her stroke diagnosis and management. A thorough ROS will help the physician further delineate the clinical characteristics of this patient's pain. This will help narrow management options. Even more critical is whether this pain is acute or chronic. Interview the patient further about how sleep, mood, and energy are either related to or separate from this pain, as these factors contribute to pain severity. The following is a guide to an interview:

   a. Onset, location, duration, character, aggravating and alleviating factors, temporal factors, current pain level, best pain, and worst pain

   b. Is there a correlation to a recent fall or relation to a specific musculoskeletal region versus dermatome?

   c. Is there a history of diabetes mellitus, carpal tunnel syndrome, low back pain, or spasticity?

   d. Past treatments used to manage the pain

   e. Current medications for pain

   f. Use of illicit drugs, alcohol, or marijuana

   g. Are there stressors at work or in the home?

2. The exam should include not only inspection and palpation of the musculoskeletal and motor system, but also testing for any sensory changes (temperature, pinprick, light touch, and pressure). Strength testing and the effort given for strength testing should be evaluated. In addition, passive and active range of motion will be important to determine if spasticity is present and associated with pain.

3. The differential diagnoses include:

   a. Central pain

   b. Orthopedic injury

   c. Carpal tunnel syndrome

   d. Cervical root impingement

   e. CRPS, type 1

   f. Vitamin deficiency

   g. Inflammatory demyelination

   h. Thyroid disease

   i. Recurrent stroke

   j. Brachial plexus dysfunction

   The suspected diagnosis is central pain syndrome based on history and exam. However, it is imperative to rule out orthopedic injuries, vitamin deficiencies, trauma, peripheral nerve impingement, and CRPS.

4. B12, folate, vitamin D, thiamine, thyroid panel, electrolytes, CMP and CBC, x-ray of the right upper extremity (RUE) and right lower extremity (RLE). NCS

and EMG studies would be helpful in excluding a PN. Triple phase bone scan might be considered if CRPS is suspected. MRI of the brain or c-spine could be considered if new abnormalities in her neuro exam were found.

5. The treatment program should include:
   a. Desensitization and strengthening with occupational therapy (OT)
   b. Topical lidocaine for transient increases in pain
   c. Start duloxetine and titrate to higher doses until pain is improved without side effects; expected side effects are discussed with patient and that the Food and Drug Administration (FDA) approved this medication for neuropathic and musculoskeletal pain.
   d. Consider alternative medications for neuropathic pain if duloxetine is not effective (amitriptyline, gabapentin, lamotrigine, carbamazepine).
   e. Optimize sleep and mood, including individual counseling.
   f. If no improvement in the above, a comprehensive pain program is recommended.

6. It is important to talk with the patient about the effects of marijuana on her cognition as well as the safety implications of her job as a bus driver. The legality of medical cannabis in individual states does not overturn the standards on alcohol, cannabis, and other drug use policies that federal, state, or private companies may require. The use of cannabis in most states that have legalized it have also mandated that it is illegal to drive while under the influence of cannabis. There is no scientific data to support its use in thalamic pain syndrome. It is also important to take time to address the patient's concerns that her mother brought up and explain that this medication is also indicated for neuropathic pain. Review with the patient that duloxetine is a safer medication for use during work or driving. It may be worthwhile to explore other medication options as well.

7. "Thank you for taking the time to talk with me about your concerns. I am really glad that you brought your concern up because this is a team effort when it comes to your medical care and your feedback is critical. Would you feel you are able to describe to me what central pain (your diagnosis) is? If not, I would like to talk about your diagnosis today and make sure that you have all the information you need about what you are being treated for. Central pain is a broader term that applies to pain syndromes in people who have had strokes, traumatic brain injuries, or other changes to their brain and spinal cord. It can show up at different times in every person's life and each person has a different experience with it depending on what caused their pain and the risk factors or medical problems they had."

"I want you to know that getting your pain managed is important, but making sure you can function daily is also a very high priority. The reason is that with central pain the goal is not to bring your pain down to zero, but rather to make sure you are able to complete your daily activities, work, sleep well, and enjoy the things you love, such as painting and drawing. Can you list out things that you want to be able to do in the next few months? We can make these individual goals to reach. Right now, you are on a low dose of duloxetine, and based on

your feedback, you have had some pain relief, but you feel like it is still interfering with your ability to function. How do you feel about increasing the dose
but also incorporating natural, evidence-based treatments such OT and/or acupuncture treatments? You also mentioned that sleep continues to be an issue
due to the pain. Have you ever tried sleep medications or supplements? There
is an over-the-counter medication called melatonin and it is a natural treatment
for sleep because your body also makes melatonin. If sleep is not optimized in
the next few weeks, I would like to suggest a cognitive behavioral talk session
with a therapist to help improve your sleep. When your sleep is not optimized
this can not only exacerbate your pain, but also make it harder to manage. Sleep
issues can also have a negative impact on your mood, metabolism, and make
you feel fatigued. If you are comfortable with this plan, then let us schedule
routine check-ins via the patient portal or here in the clinic. That way you can
update me on your progress, and we can reevaluate if the game plan should
change."

BIBLIOGRAPHY

Ferini-Strambi L. Neuropathic pain and sleep: a review. *Pain Ther.* 2017;6(1):19–23. https://doi.org/10.1007/s40122-017-0089-y

Ju ZY, Wang K, Cui HS, et al. Acupuncture for neuropathic pain in adults. *Cochrane Database Syst Rev.* 2017;(12). https://doi.org/10.1002/14651858.CD012057.pub2

Mücke M, Phillips T, Radbruch L, et al. Cannabis-based medicines for chronic neuropathic pain in adults. *Cochrane Database Syst Rev.* 2018;3(3):CD012182. https://doi.org/10.1002/14651858.CD012182.pub2

Oh H, Seo W. A comprehensive review of central post-stroke pain. *Pain Manag Nurs.* 2015;16(5):804–818. https://doi.org/10.1016/j.pmn.2015.03.002

Parekh T, Pemmasani S, Desai R. Marijuana use among young adults (18–44 years of age) and risk of stroke: a behavioral risk factor surveillance system survey analysis. *Stroke.* 2020;51(1):308–310. https://doi.org/10.1161/STROKEAHA.119.027828

Singer J, Conigliaro A, Spina E, et al. Central post stroke pain: a systematic review. *Int J Stroke.* 2017;12(4):343–355. (P4. 219). https://doi.org/10.1177/1747493017701149

Sommerfeld DK, Welmer AK. Pain following stroke, initially and at 3 and 18 months after stroke, and its association with other disabilities. *Eur J Neurol.* 2012;19:1325–1330. https://doi.org/10.1111/j.1468-1331.2012.03747.x

Abbreviations

AAC	Augmentative and alternative communication	CDT	Complete decongestive therapy
ABG	Arterial blood gas	CK	Creatine kinase
ABI	Ankle-brachial index	CMP	Comprehensive metabolic panel
ABS	Agitated Behavior Scale	CNS	Central nervous system
AC	Acromioclavicular	COPD	Chronic obstructive pulmonary disease
ACL	Anterior cruciate ligament	CPK	Creatine phosphokinase
AD	Autonomic dysreflexia	CRP	C-reactive protein
ADLs	Activities of daily living	CRPS	Complex regional pain syndrome
AFO	Ankle-foot orthosis	CRS-R	Coma Recovery Scale-Revised
ANA	Antinuclear antibody	CSF	Cerebrospinal fluid
AP	Anteroposterior	DLCO	Low diffusion for carbon monoxide
AVN	Avascular necrosis	DMII	Type II diabetes mellitus
BDI-II	Beck Depression Inventory-II	DTR	Deep tendon reflex
BLE	Bilateral lower extremities	DVT	Deep vein thrombosis
BMI	Body mass index	EDB	Extensor digiti brevis
BMP	Basic metabolic panel	EF	Ejection fraction
BP	Blood pressure	EMG	Electromyography
BPM	Beats per minute	ESR	Erythrocyte sedimentation rate
BUE	Bilateral upper extremities	FAI	Femoroacetabular impingement
CASH	Cruciform-anterior-spinal-hyperextension orthosis	FDA	Food and Drug Administration
CBC	Complete blood count	FM	Fibromyalgia
CC	Coracoclavicular		

FMLA	Family Medical Leave Act	MUPs	Motor unit potentials
GDS	Geriatric Depression Scale	MuSK	Muscle-specific tyrosine kinase
GERD	Gastroesophageal reflux disease	NCS	Nerve conduction study
GOAT	Galveston Orientation and Amnesia Test	NCV	Nerve conduction velocity
HAART	Highly active antiretroviral therapy	NP	Neuropsychological
HBI	Hypoxic brain injury	NSAIDs	Nonsteroidal anti-inflammatory drugs
HgA1c	Hemoglobin A1c	NSE	Neuron-specific enolase
HI	Homicidal ideation	OA	Osteoarthritis
HLA-B27	Human leukocyte antigen B27	O-log	Orientation-log
IBD	Inflammatory bowel disease	OT	Occupational therapy
		OTC	Over-the counter
ISCNSCI	International Standards for Neurological Classification of Spinal Cord Injury	PA	Posteroanterior
		PCA	Patient controlled anesthesia
IV	Intravenous	PCSS	Postconcussion symptom scale
LAD	Left anterior descending coronary artery	PDSA	Plan, Do, See, Act
		PEG	Percutaneous endoscopically placed gastrostomy
LDL	Low-density lipoprotein		
LOC	Loss of consciousness	PHQ	Patient Health Questionnaire
LSO	Lumbosacral orthosis	PICS	Postintensive care syndrome
MCA	Middle cerebral artery		
MCL	Medial collateral ligament	PM&R	Physical Medicine and Rehabilitation
METs	Metabolic equivalents	PN	Peripheral neuropathy
MI	Myocardial infarction	PSD	Poststroke depression
MLD	Manual lymphatic drainage	PT	Physical therapy
		PTA	Posttraumatic amnesia
MoCA	Montreal Cognitive Assessment	PVD	Peripheral vascular disease
MTSS	Medial tibial stress syndrome	RLE	Right lower extremity

ROM	Range of motion
ROS	Review of systems
RPR	Rapid plasma regain
RUE	Right upper extremity
SADQ-H	Stroke Aphasic Depression Questionnaire-Hospital Version
SARS	Severe acute respiratory syndrome
SI	Sacroiliac; Suicidal ideation
SLE	Systemic lupus erythematosus
SLP	Speech-language pathology
SNRIs	Serotonin and norepinephrine reuptake inhibitors

SOMI	Sternal occipital mandibular immobilizer
SPEP	Serum protein electrophoresis
SSNRI	Selective serotonin norepinephrine reuptake inhibitors
TBI	Traumatic brain injury
TCAs	Tricyclic antidepressants
TSH	Thyroid stimulating hormone
VA	Veterans Affairs
WBC	White blood cell
WBMRI	Whole-body magnetic resonance imaging

Index

Printed in the United States
by Baker & Taylor Publisher Services